AMAZING NATURAL MEDICINES

by Dr. Douglas Lobay, N.D.

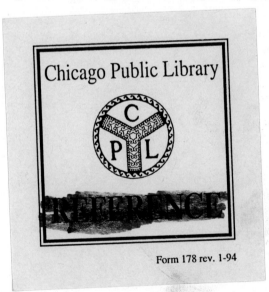

A Modern and Scientific Guide to the Use of Diet, Vitamins, Minerals and Botanical Medicines in the Treatment of Disease.

Distributed by **Gordon Soules Book**
Publishers Ltd. ● 1354-B Marine Drive,
West Vancouver BC Canada V7T 1B5
● 620-1916 Pike Place, Seattle WA 98101 US
E-mail: books@gordonsoules.com
Web site: http://www.gordonsoules.com
(604) 922 6588 Fax: (604) 688 5442

Published by
Apple Communications
Kelowna, BC

Disclaimer: The information presented here in this book is for educational purposes only and is not intended for the diagnosis and/or treatment of disease. Individuals should seek out proper medical care from licensed medical practitioners for appropriate diagnosis and treatment.

Canadian Cataloguing in Publication Data
Lobay, Doug, 1965 -
Amazing Natural Medicines

Includes Index
ISBN: 0-9695681-3-4
1. Natural Medicine 2. Naturopathy - Handbooks, manuals, etc.

Printed in Canada

TABLE OF CONTENTS

DEDICATION

To my parents for all their love and support.

ACKNOWLEDGMENTS

I would like to thank:
Mom and Dad
Arlene and Jim
Mike and Annette
Mike and Nellie
Dr. Gaetano Morello
Dr. Michael Murray
Dr. Kim Vanderlinden
Susan Carroll
Rachel and Jessica
and of course, Natalie

FOREWORD

AMAZING NATURAL MEDICINES

Amazing Natural Medicines is a modern and scientific guide to the use of diet, vitamins, minerals and botanical medicines in the treatment of common diseases. I want to present an enjoyable and informative book to educate others about the virtues of natural medicine. In the past, many conventional doctors and close-minded scientists have argued that there is no scientific basis to naturopathic medicine or the therapies that this branch of medicine employs. When I decided to attend Bastyr College of Natural Health Sciences to study naturopathic medicine, I wanted to prove to myself that naturopathic therapies were effective and that there was scientific literature to support this.

Early in my career I was fortunate enough to have Dr. Michael Murray, N.D. as a teacher and as a mentor. Dr. Murray taught botanical medicine at Bastyr College and used documented evidence from the scientific literature to support many of the claims he made. Dr. Murray along with Dr. Pizzorno wrote The Textbook of Natural Medicine the first fully referenced textbook on natural medicine written from a scientific perspective. Dr. Murray's contribution to the modern practice of naturopathic medicine is invaluable. I learned that many of the traditional methods of healing did indeed have merit and the literature abounded with research supporting many of these methods. Medical Journals like the New England Journal of Medicine and the Journal of the American Medical Association had many articles supporting natural medicine. From this foundation I began to research many of the therapies that we were taught in school. I spent countless hours at the University of Washington Medical library photocopying articles. I was surprised at the amount of documented scientific evidence for these therapies. From my research I began to write Amazing Natural Medicines.

I believe that the future of naturopathic medicine looks very bright. Natural medicine will undoubtedly play a part in modern medicine of the 21st Century. I hope you enjoy this book, Amazing Natural Medicines. Live with passion and joy.

Doug Lobay
Kelowna, B.C.

INTRODUCTION

AMAZING NATURAL MEDICINES

Naturopathic medicine is a separate and distinct branch of medicine based upon the following principles of practice:

The Healing Power of Nature (Vis Medicatrix Naturae). Vis Medicatrix Naturae acts powerfully through healing mechanisms in the body and mind to maintain and restore health. Naturopathic physicians work to restore and support these inherent healing systems when they have broken down, by using methods, medicines and techniques that are in harmony with natural processes.

First Do No Harm (Primum non nocere). Naturopathic physicians prefer non-invasive treatments which minimize the risks of harmful side effects. They are trained to know which patients they can treat safely and which ones they need to refer to other health care practitioners.

Find the Cause (Tolle Causum). Every illness has an underlying cause, often in aspects of lifestyle, diet or habits of the individual. A naturopathic physician is trained to find and remove the underlying cause of a disease.

Treat the Whole Person. Health or disease comes from a complex interaction of physical, emotional, dietary, genetic, environmental, lifestyle and other factors. Naturopathic physicians treat the whole person, taking these factors into account.

Preventive Medicine. The naturopathic approach to health care can prevent minor illnesses from developing into more serious or chronic degenerative diseases. Patients are taught the principles with which to live a healthy life; and by following these principles they can prevent most major illnesses.

HISTORY

As a distinct health care profession, Naturopathic medicine is almost 100 years old. Its roots go back through medical history to the healing wisdom of many cultures and times. At the turn of century, practioners of a variety of medical disciplines combined natural therapeutics in a way they hadn`t been combined before and joined together to form the first naturopathic medical societies. Naturopathic medical conventions in the 1920's attracted more than 10,000 practioners. Earlier in the century there were more than 20 naturopathic medical colleges and naturopathic physicians were licensed in a majority of North America.

Naturopathic medicine experienced a decline in the 1940's and 1950's with the rise and popularity of pharmaceutical drugs, technological medicine and the idea that drugs would eliminate all disease. It has experienced a resurgence in the last two decades, as a health conscious public began to seek out alternatives to conventional medicine. As a body of knowledge, naturopathic medicine continues to grow and evolve. It incorporates those elements of scientific modern medicine that forward the knowledge of the mechanisms of natural healing and therapeutics, especially in the fields of diagnosis, immunology, clinical nutrition, botanical medicine and other clinical sciences. As an organized profession, naturopathic medicine is committed to on-going research and development of its science.

THE NATUROPATHIC PHYSICIAN

Naturopathic physicians (N.D.'s) are general practitioners trained as specialists in natural medicine. They are educated in the conventional medical sciences, but they are not orthodox medical doctors (M.D.'s). Naturopathic physicians treat disease and restore health using therapies from the sciences of clinical nutrition, herbal medicine, homeopathy, physical medicine, exercise therapy, counselling. oriental medicine, acupuncture, natural childbirth and hydrotherapy. They tailor these approaches to the needs of the individual patient. Naturopathic medicine is effective in treating most health problems, whether acute or chronic. Naturopathic physicians cooperate with all other branches of medical science, referring patients to other practitioners for diagnosis or treatment when appropriate. In practice, naturopathic physicans perform physical examinations, laboratory testing, gynecological exams, nutritional and dietary assessments, metabolic analysis, allergy testing, X-ray examinations and other modern diagnostic tests. They are the only primary health care practitioners clinically trained to the needs of the individual based on a philosophy that acknowledges the patient as a participant.

The naturopathic physician has a Doctor of Naturopathic Medicine (N.D.) degree from a four year graduate level naturopathic medical college. In states and provinces where they are regulated, naturopathic physicians must pass either a national or a state/provincial level board examination and their actions are subject to review by a state/provincial Board of Examiners.

ANOTHER KIND OF DOCTOR

Naturopathic physicians are the only primary care physicians clinically trained in a wide variety of medical systems. Some of the natural therapies practiced by naturopathic physicians are:

Clinical Nutrition. Nutrition and the therapeutic use of foods have always been a cornerstone of naturopathic medicine. A growing body of scientific knowledge in this area is reflected in numerous professional journals of nutrition and dietary sciences, validating the naturopathic approach to diet and nutrition. Many medical conditions can be treated as effectively with foods and nutritional supplements as they can be by any other means, but with fewer complications and side effects. Naturopathic physicians receive more than 140 classroom hours in clinical nutrition, while in contrast most medical doctors receive fewer than 20 hours.

Homeopathic Medicine. This powerful system of medicine is more than 200 years old and is widely accepted in other countries around the world. The Royal Family of England uses a homeopathic physician. Homeopathic medicines act to strengthen the body's innate immune response; they seldom have side effects. Some conditions that conventional medicine has no effective treatment for, respond well to homeopathy.

Botanical Medicine. Many plant substances are powerful medicines, with advantages over conventional drugs. They are effective and safe when used properly, in the right dose and in the proper combinations with other herbs and treatments. A resurgence of scientific research in Europe and Asia is demonstrating that some plant substances are superior to synthetic drugs used in clinical situations. Naturopathic physicians are trained in both the art and the science of botanical medicine.

Physical Medicine. In the last 100 years, various methods of applying treatments through the manipulation of the muscles, bones and spine have been developed in North America. Naturopathic Medicine has its own techniques, collectively known as naturopathic manipulative therapy. Physical medicine also includes, but is not limited to, physiotherapy using heat and cold, gentle electric pulses, ultrasound, diathermy, hydrotherapy and exercise therapy.

Natural Childbirth. Some Naturopathic physicians provide natural childbirth care in an out-of-hospital setting. They offer pre-natal and post-natal care using the most modern diagnostic techniques. When natural childbirth is not medically indicated, because of high risk, patients are referred for appropriate care.

Oriental Medicine. Naturopathic physicians are trained in the fundamentals of oriental medicine and diagnosis and many use acupuncture, acupressure and oriental botanical medicine in their practices.

Counselling and Stress Management. Mental attitudes and emotional states can be important elements in healing and disease. Naturopathic physicians are trained in various psychological techniques, including counselling, nutritional balancing, stress management, hypnotherapy, biofeedback and other methods.

Minor Surgery. This includes repair of superficial wounds, removal of foreign bodies, cysts and other superficial masses with local anaesthesia as needed.

21st CENTURY BOTANICAL MEDICINE

Botanical medicine is experiencing a renaissance in Europe and North America. The modern use of plants and plant derivatives in the treatment of disease is being validated by scientific research. The World Health Organization (WHO) has estimated that 80% of the world population of 5 billion relies on traditional medicines for their primary health care needs. Over 25% of all prescription drugs in North America have contained active constituents derived from plants. One of the great fallacies and misconceptions being perpetuated by the medical establishment is that natural therapies, including botanical medicine, have no valid scientific proof. One of the goals of this book is to dispel the myths and skepticism surrounding natural medicine, including botanical medicine, and bridge the gap between folk medicine and modern science.

There are many advantages of using botanical medicines. As a rule of thumb, botanical medicines are less toxic than their synthetic counterparts and offer less risk of adverse effects. Botanical preparations consists of many synergistic factors that act together, demonstrating that the whole plant or crude plant extract is superior to the action of the isolated constituent. The mechanism of action of many botanical medicines is to correct the underlying cause of dysfunction. Botanical medicines are often cheaper than their synthetic counterparts.

Traditionally the pharmaceutical industry has paid little attention to the herbal industry. Since a plant or botanical preparation cannot be patented and no profit generated, little research has been done on traditional herbal medicines. However, don't be mislead, botanical medicine is a powerful and effective medicine. Botanical medicines contain many pharmacologically active chemical constituents. One of the problems in the herbal industry has been the lack of quality control. There has been no way of ensuring the quality of an herbal product the consumer is using. Substitutions, adulterants and misrepresentations have been widespread in the herbal industry. Fortunately, in Asia and Europe several pharmaceutical firms became re-interested in traditional herbal medicine and a new chapter in botanical medicine was opened. Through modern technology new techniques became available to measure and quantify the active chemical constituents in many plants. Active chemical constituents responsible for the pharmacolgical action of many plants once used widely in folk medicine were identified for the first time. New techniques including thin-layer chromatography (TLC) and high-pressure liquid chromatography (HPLC) are now being used to isolate and quantify active constituents. Additionally, improvements in cultivation, harvesting, curing procedures, storage, shelf life added to the resurgence of this field. Standardized botanical extracts containing a specified quantity of active chemicals responsible for specific pharmacologic effects are now available.

Let's use Ginseng as an example. Ginseng is one of the most popular herbs in the market place and is widely used for its tonifying and tranquilizing effects. There have been many different ginseng preparations commercially available in the market place. Modern technology has been responsible for the identification and isolation of chemicals in the crude plant responsible for its reported therapeutic actions. Ginsenosides are a group of chemically related compounds responsible for the therapeutic effects of ginseng. The usual concentration of ginsenosides in ginseng root has been determined to range from 2.0 to 5.0%. Using modern technological procedures, high quality ginseng extracts are now available guaranteeing a specific concentration of active ginsenosides (i.e. 5.0% ginsenoside content by weight).

Another major improvement in botanical preparations has been in the area of extraction and concentration. By knowing the active chemical constituents in herbal preparations, an effort was made to concentrate these constituents to produce a high potency preparation. These high potency preparations are typically produced from four times the quantity of the original herbal material. A 4:1 concentration means that 4 parts of the crude herbal extract is equivalent to one part of the concentrated standardized extract. Again to use ginseng as an example; in concentrated preparations the active ginsenosides are concentrated above and beyond the range that they are normally found in the original plant. Preparations containing 14% ginsenosides have been produced.New and improved botanical medicines containing specified amounts of active chemical constituents are being produced as standardized herbal extracts. Also, improvements in the study of the toxic side effects of botanical medicines has paralleled the improvement in the quality of botanical medicines being produced.

The future of natural medicine, including botanical medicine, has entered a new and exciting era. The therapeutic value of natural medicine is being validated by scientific research. The future of natural medicine, including botanical medicine looks very bright and undoubtedly will play a major part of medicine in the 21st century.

REFERENCES

(1) American Association of Naturopathic Physicians (AANP) brochure, Naturopathic Medicine: What it is...What it can do for you, Seattle, Washington.

CHAPTER 1

BOOSTING YOUR IMMUNE SYSTEM

The human body has an incredible innate ability to heal itself and resist infection from bacteria, fungi and viruses. The capacity of the body to resist disease and infection is called immunity. This innate ability makes the body resistant to such diseases as polio, cholera, syphilis, mumps and measles, which are very destructive and even lethal to the human being. In addition to its innate immunity the human body has the ability to develop extremely powerful specific immunity against individual invading agents such as lethal bacteria, viruses and toxins. This developed immunity is called acquired immunity. Acquired immunity consists of two basic closely allied types: cell-mediated immunity and antibody-mediated immunity. Cell-mediated immunity consists of large number of white blood cells that actively seek out and destroy foreign material. Antibody-mediated immunity consists of protein molecules that bind and promote the destruction of foreign material. The immune system is an exceedingly complex and responsive system that helps us to resist infection. There are safe and natural alternatives to stimulate immune function and optimize health.

DIET

Diet plays a very important role in all aspects of immune function. Manipulation of dietary factors has been shown to optimize immune response. Adequate dietary protein is necessary for proper immune function. (1) Excessive intake of fats, including cholesterol and polyunsaturated fats is associated with immuno-depression. (2) Sugar impairs all aspects of immune function and should be avoided. Sugar intake has been shown to impair cell-mediated immunity, antibody-mediated immunity and the ability of cells to engulf and digest foreign material. (3)

NUTRIENTS

A modest increase in dietary intake of Vitamin A, enhances immune response while excessive doses depresses immune response. (1) Supplementation with Beta-carotene stimulates immune function and has been shown to increase helper T-cells. (4)

B-complex deficiencies have been correlated with decreased antibody production and impairs cell-mediated immunity. (2) Deficiencies of Riboflavin (Vitamin B2), Vitamin B-12, Pantothenic acid and Folic acid impair immune function. Pyridoxine (Vitamin B6) is required for normal nucleic acid, protein synthesis and cell division. Pyridoxine deficiency has a profound effect on immune function and has been shown to affect both cell-mediated immunity and antibody-mediated immunity. (5)

Vitamin C deficiency impairs immune function and the ability of cells to engulf and digest foreign material. Vitamin C supplementation increases antibody levels and has been shown to improve immune function in the elderly and may suppress the symptoms associated with acquired immune deficiency syndrome (AIDS). (2, 6)

Vitamin D deficiency has been shown to depress immune function. (7)

Vitamin E deficiency has also been shown to depress immune function and supplementation enhances immune response. (8)

Copper deficiency has been correlated with increased incidence of infection and diminished cell-mediated immune response. (2)

Iodine deficiency has been associated with impaired bacteriocidal activity of white blood cells. (20)

Iron deficiency and excessive iron intake may impair immune function. (2) Magnesium deficiency impairs antibody production. (1)

Selenium deficiency especially along with Vitamin E deficiency has been shown to impair cell-mediated immunity and may also impair antibody-mediated immunity. (1)

Zinc deficiency impairs immune function, while moderate doses of zinc supplements has been shown to stimulate the immune system. (2) However, excessive doses of zinc may impair immune response. (9)

L-carnitine supplementation may benefit immune function and supplementation with dimethylglycine (DMG) may enhance both antibody and cell-mediated immunity. (10, 11) Deficiencies involving any of the essential amino acids have been shown to depress immune function. (2)

Essential fatty acids are required for optimal immune function. Supplementation with Omega-6 oil may be beneficial. Omega-6 oil has been shown to enhance the synthesis of prostaglandin E1, which plays an important role on the regulation of T-cell function. (2)

Taurine supplementation has also been shown to increase immune response and the ability of cells to engulf and digest foreign material. (12)

Cadmium, lead and mercury toxicities impair immune function and may cause severe immuno-depression. (13)

BOTANICAL MEDICINES

Astragalus root (Astragalus membranaceous) is one of the most popular herbal medicines in China and Asia. Slices of the root resemble popsicle sticks or tongue depressors and are distributed widely in chinese pharmacies and herbal stores. The herb is noted for tonifying and immune stimulating activity. Scientific research is beginning to confirm some of the folklore use of this popular herb. Large weight polysaccharides are believed to be responsible for the immune stimulating activity. Astragalus extracts have been used in several studies to treat immune deficiencies creating by chronic disease and cancer. Astragalus boosts natural interferon levels and enhances certain aspects of cell-mediated immunity. (14,15,16)

Maitake mushroom (Grifola frondosa) is widely consumed as a culinary delight and medicinal tonic throughout parts of Asia including China and Japan. Large molecular weight polysaccharide found in small amounts in the mushroom mycelia are believed to be responsible for the purported immune stimulating activity of this plant. Purified extracts containing the polysaccharhide derivatives, specifically the 1,3 beta-D-glucan, enhance certain aspects of cell-mediated immunity including both macrophages and T-cells. Maitake extract have demonstrated anti-tumour activity in certain types of cancers. Maitake extracts also lower cholesterol and reduce elevated blood sugar levels. (17,18,19)

Shitake mushroom (Lentinus edodes) is another culinary delight consumed by Asians and has reported immune stimulating activity. The lipopolysaccharide derivatives of Shitake mycelia, specifically a mannose monomer called lentinan, enhance certain aspects of cell-mediated immunity including both macrophages, tumour necrosis factor and T-cell activation. Shitake extracts have demonstrated anti-tumour activity in certain types of cancer. Additionally, Shitake has been reported to lower blood pressure and elevated cholesterol levels. (20,21,22)

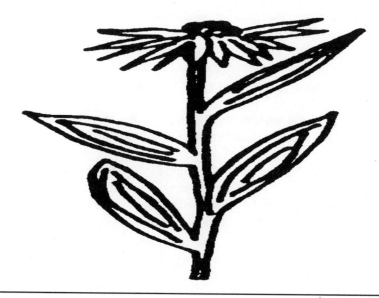

Purple coneflower (Echinacea angustifolia)

Purple coneflower (Echinacea angustifolia) is a perennial flower native to the Great Plains of North America that grows from 20 to 100 centimeters in height. Echinacea was one of the most widely used medicinal plant of the Plain Indians who used Echinacea to treat toothaches, coughs, colds, sore throats, snakebites and as a painkiller. Recent scientific research, mostly by German researchers, has shown that Echinacea has remarkable immune stimulation properties.(23)

Many active ingredients have been identified in Echinacea and it appears that they work synergistically. Echinacoside, a glycoside, comprising approximately 1.0% of the dry weight of Echinacea, possesses mild antibiotic activity. Echinacin, a polysaccharide sugar, has immune stimulating and antiviral activity. Echinacin has been shown to consist of two polysaccharides; polysaccharide A and polysaccharide B. (24) Echinacin, a polysaccharide in Echinacea, inhibits the activity of the enzyme hyaluronidase which is responsible for the breakdown of connective tissue.

Echinacea enhances connective tissue stabilization by inhibiting the hyaluronidase enzyme. Connective tissue and ground substance forms a barrier between cells, thereby inhibiting invasion by infectious micro-organisms and decreasing inflammation. Echinacin B has been shown to combine with hyaluronidase, temporarily inactivating it and thus promotes connective tissue integrity. It has been suggested that other constituents in Echinacea may be involved in connective tissue stabilization in addition to echinacin. Echinacea enhances wound healing by stimulating connective tissue regeneration. (25)

Echinacea stimulates the breakdown of fibrin from clots into polysaccharides which are transformed into new connective tissue. (26)

Echinacea stimulates the immune system by enhancing macrophage function. Echinacin has demonstrated to activate macrophages to engulf and destroy invading foreign organisms. In addition, echinacin binds membrane receptors on the surface of T-lymphocytes. This facilitates the production of the intercellular messengers, interferon and other lymphokines which further activate macrophages and natural killer cells. (27)

Echinacin further activates the complement pathway of the immune system. The complement pathway involves a complex series of enzymatic reactions in normal blood that involve proteins and antigen-antibody complexes. Complement proteins bind antigen-antibody complexes which enhances the destruction of foreign material. Echinacin also increases properdin, an enzymatic protein involved in the alternate complement pathway. (28) Echinacin stimulates a non-specific immune response that increases the function of macrophages, T-lymphocyes and the complement pathway.

Echinacea extracts have also demonstrated antiviral activity against influenza, herpes and vesicular stomatitis viruses. The antiviral activity of Echinacea extracts is believed to be related to the plant's non-specific immune modulating activity. Connective tissue stabilization and regeneration and direct activation of macrophages and T-lymphocytes are among the immune modulating effects of Echinacea. (29)

Clinically, Echinacea has been used to treat various bacteria caused skin infections with good results. Echinacea stimulates production of white blood cells in the bone marrow of patients undergoing radiation therapy. (30) In 203 patients with chronic recurrent vaginal infection, a combination of Echinacea cream and liquid extract proved very effective in eliminating the infection and preventing further infections. (31) Further clinical research into the immune stimulating actions of Echinacea is necessary to support its use as an immune stimulator.

Echinacea is safe and non-toxic. There appears to be no side effects with long term use and its use during pregnancy remains unknown. (24)

RECOMMENDATIONS: Daily unless otherwise stated.

Vitamin A..50,000-100,000 IU
Beta-carotene..200 mg
Vitamin B-complex...50-100 mg
Folic Acid..400-800 mcg
Pantothenic Acid...500 mg
Vitamin B6..25-50 mg
Vitamin B2..10-25 mg
Vitamin B12..100 mcg
Vitamin C...1000-3000 mg
Vitamin D...400-800 IU
Vitamin E...400-800IU
Copper...2-4 mg

Iodine..100-200 mcg
Iron..10-25 mg
Magnesium..400-800 mg
Selenium...400-800 mcg
Zinc..25-50 mg
Carnitine...500 mg
Dimethylglycine...200 mg
Essential amino acids...3-6 gm
Essential fatty acids..3-6 gm
Astragalus membranaceous...............................500-1000 mg
Maitake extract...250-500 mg
Shitake extract...250-500 mg
Echinacea angustifolia (6.5:1)...........................500-1000 mg

REFERENCES

(1) Levy JA: Nutrition and the immune system. Basic and Clinical Immunology, 4th edition. Lange Medical Publications, Los Altos, CA.,pp. 297-305, 1982

(2) Chandra RK: Nutrition and immunity - Basic considerations. Part 1. Contemp. Nutr. 11(11), 1986

(3) Bernstein J et al: Depression of lymphocytic transformation following oral glucose ingestion. Am. J. Clin. Nutr. 30:613, 1977

(4) Alexander M et al: Oral beta-carotene can increase the number of OKT4 cells in human blood. Immunology Letters 9:221-24, 1985

(5) Axelrod AE et al: Relationship of pyridoxine to immunological phenomena. Vitam. Horm. 22:591-607, 1964

(6) Kennes B et al: Effect of vitamin C supplements on cell-mediated immunity in old people. Gerontology 29(5):305-10, 1983

(7) Toss G et al: Delayed hypersensitivity response and vitamin D deficiency. Int. J. Vit. Nutr. Res. 53(1):27-31, 1983

(8) Beisel WR et al: Single-nutrient effects on immunolgic functions. JAMA 245(1):53-58, 1981

(9) Chandra RK: Excessive intake of zinc impairs immune responses. JAMA 252:1443-46, 1985

(10) Se Simone C et al: Vitamins and Immunity: Influence of L-carnitine on the immune system. Acta Vitaminol. Enzymol. 4(1-2):135-40, 1982

(11) Graber CD et al: Immunomodulating properties of dimethylglycine in humans. J. Infectious Dis. 143(1):101-5, 1981

(12) Masuda M et al: Influences of taurine on functions of rat neutrophils. Jap. J. Pharmacol. 34(1):116-118, 1984

(13) Halstead BW: Immune augmentation therapy. J. Int. Acad. Prevent. Med. 9(1):5-19, 1985

(14)   Chu DT et al: Immunotherapy with Chinese medicinal herbs. II. Reversal of cyclophosphamide-induced immune suppression by administration of fractionated Astragalus membranaceous in vivo. J Clin Lab Immunol, 25(3):125-9 1988 Mar
(15)   Weng XS: Treatment of leucopenia with pure Astragalus preparation — an analysis of 115 leucopenic cases. Chunh Kuo Chung Ksi I Chieh Ho Tsa Chih, 15(8): 462-4, 1996 Aug
(16)   Zhao XZ: Effects of Astragalus membranaceus on natural killer cell activity of peripheral blood mononuclear in systemic lupus eruthematosus. Chung Kuo Chung Hsi I Chieh Ho Tsa Chih, 12(11):669-71, 645 1192 Nov
(17)   Suzuki K et al: Effect of a polysaccharide fraction from Grofola frodosa on immune response in mice. J Pharmacobiodyn, 8(3):217-26, 1985 Mar
(18)   Takeyama T et al: Host-mediated antitumor effect of grifolan NMF-5N, a polysaccharide obtained from Grifola frondosa. J Pharmacobiodyn, 10(11):644-51, 1987 Nov
(19)   Suzuki I et al: Antitumor and immunomodulating activities of a beta-glucan obtained from liquid-cultures Grifola frondosa. Chem Pharm Bull (Tokyo), 37(2):410-3, 1989 Feb
(20)   Wang GL and Lin ZB: The immunomodulatory effect of lentinan. Yas Hsueh Pao, 31(2):86-90, 1996
(21)   Kosaka A et al: Effect of lentinan administration of adrenalectomized rats and patiens with breast cancer. Gan To Kagaku Ryoho, 9(8):1474-81, 1982 Aug
(22)   Taguchi T: Effects of lentinan in advanced or recurent cases of gastric, colorectal and breast cancer. Gan To Kagaku Ryoho, 10(2 Pt 2):387-93, 1983 Feb
(23)   Kindscher K: Ethnobotany of Purple coneflower (Echinacea angustifolia, Asteraceae) and other Echinacea species. Ethnobotany 43(4):498-507, 1989
(24)   Wagner H et al: Immunostimulatory Drugs of Fungi and Higher Plants. Economic and Medicinal Plant Research Vol. I:113-153 Academic PressNew York, NY, 1985
(25)   Tyler V et al: Pharmacognosy, 8th edition. Lea & Febiger, Philadelphia, Pennsylvania, 1981
(26)   Koch E et al: Experimental studies concerning the local action of echinacea angustifolia and e. purpurea. Arzneim. Forsch. 3:16-19, 1953
(27)   Stimpel M et al: Macrophage and Induction of Macrophage Cytotoxicity by Purified Polysaccharide Fractions from the Plant Echinacea purpurea. Infection and Immunity46(3):845-9, 1984
(28)   Mose J: Effect of echinacin on phagocytosis and natural killer cells. Med. Welt. 34:1463-7, 1983
(29)   Wacker A et al: Virus-inhibition by echinacea purpurea. Planta Medica 33:89-102, 1978
(30)   Foster S: Echinacea Exalted. Ozark Beneficial Plant Project, Missouri, p. 23, 1985
(31)   Coeungniet E: Empiricism-Echinacea. Eclectic Medical Journal. 57(8):421-427, 1897

CHAPTER 2

BUILDING HEALTHY BONES

Osteoporosis is a disease that has reached epidemic proportions in North America. Osteoporosis affects over 20 million individuals in North America each year. It accounts for more than 1 million fractures per year in people over the age of 45 years. The most common osteoporotic related fractures are to the wrist, back and hip. Hip fractures are by the most serious consequence of osteoporosis. About 20% of those individuals who sustain a hip fracture die with within one year because of complications such as blood clots or pneumonia. The estimated health costs of osteoporotic related fractures in North America is close to $10 billion dollars per year. With an ever increasing geriatric population the search for a cure to this disease is of paramount importance. Osteoporosis is defined as decreased bone density. Osteoporosis literally means "porous bone." Bone mass decreases and bones become deteriorated and porous. Osteoporotic bone is prone to fractures with a minimal amount of stress. Some bone loss appears to be a normal consequence of aging. However, excessive bone loss is considered to be pathological.

Osteoporosis is an insidious disease. By the time clinical symptoms appear there has been a significant amount of bone loss. At the early stage of this disease there are no apparent signs and symptoms. By the time standard X-rays begin to show bone loss at least 30 to 40% of bone mass has already been lost. Pain is probably the most common symptom associated with this condition. Bone fractures can cause a significant amount of pain and discomfort. Chronic pain due to muscle spasm may persist long after osteoporotic bone fractures have healed. In some osteoporotic individuals anterior wedging of thoracic vertebra causes loss of height and the formation of the characteristic "hump-back." In other individuals the initial symptom of osteoporosis is severe pain in the mid-back. Severe mid-back pain can indicate an acute compression or wedge fracture of a vertebral body between the levels of the eight thoracic vertebra to the second lumbar vertebra. In other individuals a fracture of radial bone near the wrist called a Colle's fracture is the first sign of this disease.   In yet other individuals a fracture of the hip bone is the first sign that osteoporosis exists

Standard medical treatment of osteoporosis focuses on pharmacologic hormone therapy. Most conventional medical doctors recommend estrogen therapy to treat or prevent osteoporosis. Estrogen is a naturally occurring hormone that is produced in the female ovaries throughout reproductive life.   At the onset of menopause the ovaries stop functioning and the production of estrogen diminishes.   Estrogen has been clearly shown to reduce bone loss by about 50% in menopausal women.   Estrogen is quite effective in slowing bone loss by reducing bone breakdown and reabsorption.   Although the effectiveness of estrogen therapy at menopause is well established , it is not clear what benefits, if any, derive from instituting estrogen therapy ten years or more after menopause

One of the toughest decisions a women makes in her life is whether or not to take hormone replacement therapy.   There are pros and cons for hormone replacement therapy.   The main negative effects of this therapy are due the adverse side effects of estrogen. Adverse side effects of estrogen therapy include nausea, vomiting, headaches, high blood pressure, jaundice, gallstones, fluid retention, swelling, edema, blood sugar abnormalities, blood clots, thrombophlebitis, breast pain, fibrocystic breast disease, breast cancer, fibroids, endometriosis, endometrial cancer and uterine cancer.   The most serious side effect of estrogen therapy in post-menopausal women is the risk of estrogen sensitive cancers such as breast and uterine cancer.   The lowest daily dose found to generally effective is 0.625 milligrams of conjugated estrogens, such as Premarin.   A typical dosing schedule of Premarin is 0.625 milligrams per day on days 1 through 25 of the female reproductive cycle.   Other research indicates that when combined with 1000 milligrams of calcium, 0.3 milligrams of conjugated estrogens is equally effective. (1,2,3)

DIET

A strong relationship between dietary habits and the development of osteoporosis is beginning to emerge.   What you eat can will affect how strong and healthy your bones are.   A diet high in animal protein has been associated with increased risk of osteoporosis. Scientific studies have demonstrated that excessive consumption of animal protein can produce bone loss. Increased consumption of protein is known to increase urine calcium loss. The by-product of protein breakdown in the body is acidic residues. Calcium is used by the body to buffer the effects of acids. Calcium is reabsorbed from bones and travels into the blood where it helps to neutralize these acids. Calcium is then excreted through the urine. Demographic studies demonstrate that those countries and cultures with the highest per capita protein consumption, also have the highest rate of osteoporosis. (1,9)

A diet high in sugar and refined carbohydrates has been associated with increased risk of osteoporosis. In the 1800's the average per person sugar consumption was about 10 to 12 pounds per year. Today in the 1990's the average per person sugar consumption has increased dramatically to 139 pounds per year. This translates to about 41 teaspoons of sugar per day for the average person. Increased consumption of sugar increases urinary calcium loss. Increased sugar consumption has demonstrated a cortisone-like thinning effect on bone tissue. Additionally refined sugar is usually devoid of any nutritional value. Sugar and other refined foods have little or no vitamin and mineral content. This means as we eat more sugar, we are getting less vitamins and minerals. Less nutrients leads to the development of osteoporosis. (1,10)

A diet high in caffeine containing foods and beverages such as coffee, tea, soda pop and chocolate has been associated with increased risk of osteoporosis. Increased consumption of caffeine containing foods leads to increased urinary calcium loss. Those individuals with the highest daily caffeine consumption had the highest calcium urine loss. Additionally, those individuals with the highest caffeine consumption were more likely to sustain a hip fracture. (1,11)

Excessive consumption of alcohol is associated with increased risk of osteoporosis. Chronic, habitual drinkers are known to at high risk for developing osteoporosis. The effect of alcohol on bones is not completely understood. However, large doses of alcohol can increase calcium loss in the urine. Additionally, poor dietary habits and nutritional deficiencies are common among chronic alcoholics. The effects of small to moderate doses of alcohol on bones is not known at this time. (1,12)

A diet high in phosphorus has been associated with increased development of osteoporosis. High phosphorus foods include animal protein, dairy, cheese and soda pops. Phosphorus is known to combine with calcium to form complexes that are excreted through the urine. Also, the foods high in phosphorus are high in protein and caffeine, which may further contribute to bone loss. (1,13

VITAMINS AND MINERALS

Calcium deficiency is one of the most common mineral deficiencies in North America. Calcium deficiency is one of the main factors in the development of weak bones and osteoporosis. Symptoms of calcium deficiency include muscle cramps, especially during exercise and pregnancy, muscle spasms, muscle tetany, bone pain, fractures that won't heal, poor blood clotting, menstrual cramps, low back pain and insomnia. (1, 2, 14, 15)

Vitamin B6 or pyridoxine is required to make strong connective tissue and bone. Vitamin B6 is used to crosslink connective tissue fibers before they are made into bone. Crosslinking helps to make bones strong and durable. Vitamin B6 is also used in the liver to help break down toxic substances that can contribute to the development of osteoporosis. Vitamin B6 deficiency can cause osteoporosis. Vitamin B6 deficiency is more common in North America. (1,16)

Folic acid is required to inactivate toxins that are produced in the body which can cause osteoporosis. Homocysteine is a toxic by-product of protein metabolism in the human body. Homocysteine can can cause weaken bones and lead to osteoporosis. The liver normally converts homocysteine into harmless by-products. Folic acid is necessary to help convert homocysteine into less toxic chemicals. Folic acid deficiency can impair the body's ability to inactivate homocysteine and other such toxins. Folic acid deficiency occurs much more commonly than is generally realized. Poor dietary habits, high fat diet, smoking, excessive alcohol consumption and oral contraceptive use can can lead to folic acid deficiency. (1,17)

Vitamin C is necessary for proper bone and connective tissue development. Vitamin C is required for crosslinking of connective tissue fiber. The established RDA for vitamin C is 60 milligrams per day for an adult. Vitamin C deficiency can cause osteoporosis. Marginal vitamin C intake can impair proper bone development. (1,18)

Vitamin D is necessary for proper calcium absorption in the intestines. Vitamin D also prevents loss of calcium in urine through the kidneys. Vitamin D deficiency can lead to decreased calcium absorption and to the development of osteoporosis. Sunshine is necessary for the conversion of inactive vitamin D to the the active form. Lack of sunshine, especially in winter time in northern climates, can lead to vitamin D deficiency. Other factors that contribute to vitamin D deficiency include lack of dietary intake and malabsorption. (1,2)

Vitamin K is required for the production of osteocalcin, a protein found in bone. Osteocalcin provides the framework on which calcium is deposited to form solid bone. Vitamin K deficiency leads to decreased osteocalcin production, decreased calcium deposition and osteoporosis. Vitamin K deficiency results from decreased dietary intake and malabsorption. Bacteria in the large intestine manufacture vitamin K. However, frequent use of antibiotics can kill these beneficial bacteria and can further contribute to vitamin K deficiency. (1,19)

Boron is one of the lesser known trace minerals whose function in human nutrition is just beginning to be understood. Boron is required to activate steroid hormones, primarily estrogen to its more active forms. It may also be necessary to activate vitamin D to its active form. No RDA for boron has been established. Current research indicates that the daily requirement is probably 1 to 3 milligrams per day. Fruits, vegetables and nuts are the main dietary sources of boron. Boron appears to be relatively non-toxic and few side effects have been reported. (1,20)

Copper is necessary for the crosslinking of connective tissue. Also copper supplementation may help to decrease bone breakdown. Copper deficiency leads to reduced bone strength. The current RDA for copper is 2 milligrams per day. (1,21)

Magnesium plays an important role in bone development. Magnesium activates certain bone forming enzymes and it activates vitamin D to its active form. Magnesium deficiency contributes to abnormal bone development and osteoporosis. Magnesium deficiency commonly occurs throughout North America. (1,23)

Manganese is a trace mineral that is required for proper bone and connective tissue development. Manganese helps to mineralize bone and improves overall bone density. Managanese deficiency can cause bones to weak and of poor density. Manganese deficiency occurs more commonly than is generally realized. (1,22)

Silicon is a mineral that is necessary to make healthy bones, ligaments, tendons, hair and nails. Silicon is used to crosslink connective tissue fibers. Crosslinking helps to make connective tissue, including bone, strong and durable. Silicon deficiency leads to abnormal bone development. No RDA for silicon has been established. Silicon appears to quite safe for long term use. (1,24)

Strontium is a lesser known trace mineral that occurs in relatively large amounts in bones and teeth. The exact function of strontium in making healthy bones is not known. Current research indicates that strontium helps to decrease bone breakdown. Strontium occurs in many different foods. It is not known whether or not strontium deficiency occurs. Strontium supplementation in osteoporotic patients significantly reduced bone degeneration and markedly reduced bone pain. No RDA for strontium has been established. Strontium appears to be safe for long term use. (1,25)

Zinc is essential for normal bone formation. Zinc enhances to the action of vitamin D. Zinc deficiency can contribute to the development of osteoporosis. Zinc deficiency occurs much more commonly than is generally realized. (1,26)

RECOMMENDATIONS: Daily unless otherwise stated

Vitamin B-complex ....50 mg
Vitamin B6...25 to 50 mg
Folic acid...400-800 mcg
Vitamin C..100-200 mg
Vitamin D..200-400 IU
Vitamin K..100-300 mcg
Boron..1-3 mg
Calcium..1000-2000 mg
Copper...1-3 mg
Manganese...10-30 mg

Magnesium..400-750 mg
Silicon..1-3 mg
Strontium..500-1000 mcg
Zinc..10-30 mg

REFERENCES

(1) Gaby, Alan R: Preventing and Reversing Osteoporosis, Prima Publishing, Rocklin, CA, 1994

(2) Watts, Nelson B: Osteoporosis, American Family Physician, pp. 193-207, November 1988

(3) Guyton A C: Textbook of Medical Physiology, W.B. Saunders, Philadelphia, PA, 1985

(4) Raisz, Lawrence G: Biochemical Markers of Bone Turnover: A new Approach in Osteoporosis, Osteoporosis Report, Washington, D.C., Spring 1994

(5) Aloia A, et al: Risk Factors for Postmenopausal Osteoporosis, American Journal of Medicine, 78:95-100, 1985

(6) Follingstad, A H: Estriol, the forgotten estrogen, JAMA, 239:29-30

(7) Prior, J C: Progesterone as a bone-trophic hormone, Endocrinol Rev., 11:386-398

(8) Yeater R and Martin R: Senile Osteoporosis: The effects of execise, Postgrad. Med., 75:147-9, 1984

(9) Licata A, et al: Acute effects of dietary protein on calcium metabolism in patients with osteoporosis, J. Gerontol., 36:14-9, 1981

(10) Thom J, et al: The influence of refined carbohydrates on urinary calcium excretion, Brit. J. Urol., 50:459-64, 1978

(11) Hollingery P W, et al: Effect of dietary caffeine and aspirin on urinary calcium and hydroxyproline excretion in pre and postmenopausal women, Fed. Proc., 44:1149

(12) Spencer H, et al: Alcohol-osteoporosis, Am. J. Clin. Nutr., 41:847

(13) Heaney RP and Recker RR: Effects of nitrogen, phosphorus and caffeine on calcium balance in women, J. Lab. Clin. Med., 99:46-55, 1982

(14) Dunne, Lavone J: Nutrition Almanac, third edition, McGraw-Hill Inc., New York, NY, 1990

(15) Lee CJ, et al: Effects of supplementation of diets with calcium and calcium-rich foods on bone density in elderly females with osteoporosis, Am. J. Clin. Nutr., 34:819-23, 1981

(16) Ellis JM and Presley J: Vitamin B6: The doctor's report, Harper and Row, New York, NY, pp. 39-73, 1973

(17) Brattstrom LE, et al: Folic acid responsive postmenopausal homocysteinemia, Metabol., 34:1073-7,1985

(18) Hyams DE and Ross EJ: Scurvy, megaloblastic anemia and osteoporosis, Brit. J. Clin. Pract., 17:332-40, 1963

(19) Gallop PM, et al: Carboxylated calcium-binding proteins and vitamin K, New Engl. J. Med., 302:1460-66, 1980

(20) Nielsen FH, et al: Boron enhances and mimics some of the effects of estrogen

therapy in postmenopausal women, J. Trace Elem. Exp. Med., 5:237-46,1992

(21) Wilson TJ, et al: Inhibition of active bon resorption by copper, Calcif. Tissue Int., 33:35-39, 1981

(22) Raloff J: Reasons for boning up on manganese, Science News, 130:199, September, 1986

(23) Cohen L and Kitzes R: Infrared spectroscopy and magnesium content of bone mineral in osteoporotic women, Isr. J. Med. Sci., 17:1123-25, 1981

(24) Carlisle EM: Silicon localization and calcification in developing bone, Fed. Proc., 28:374, 1969

(25) Skoryna SC: Effects of oral supplementation with stable strontium, Can. Med. Assoc., 125:703-12, 1981

(26) Atik OS: Zinc and sneile osteoporosis, J. American Geriat. Soc., 31:790-91, 1983

CHAPTER 3

CLEARING BLADDER INFECTIONS

Urinary tract infections are a common infection of the urinary tract and typically involves the ureters, bladder and urethra and in more serious cases, the kidneys. Urinary tract infections (UTIs) are experienced by 10 to 20% of the population with a much higher prevalence in females than in males and have a high rate of re-occurrence. Lower urinary tract infections commonly involve the bladder causing cystitis and is characterized by difficult or painful urination and increased urgency and increased frequency of urination. Fever, chills and flank pain usually accompany the other complaints. In more serious cases, symptoms include blood in urine, diarrhea, vomiting and kidney dysfunction. The association of urinary tract infections with sexual intercourse in women is known as "honeymoon cystitis" and infection usually follows sexual intercourse within 24 hours. Infection will recur in up to 50% of patients within one year following treatment. Urine is usually sterile and infections are usually caused by the bacteria, E.coli, which accounts for 80 to 90% of UTIs. Safe and effective natural therapies are available for the treatment of urinary tract infections.

DIET

Individuals with urinary tract infections should drink copious amounts of fluids, primarily as water. Increased consumption of water increases urination and flushes the urinary tract of bacteria. (1) Cranberry juice from the berries of Vaccinium macrocarpon has been used since the mid-1800's to lower urinary pH and effectively treat urinary tract infections. It is believed that cranberries, prunes and plums contain benzoic acid or some related compound that the body metabolizes into hippuric acid; a bacteriostatic agent in high concentrations. Cranberry juice contain 88% water, anthocyanin dyes, catechin, triterpenoids, about 10% carbohydrates and small amounts of protein. (2) A high fluid intake must accompany ingestion of cranberry juice to achieve relief from urinary tract infections. Hippuric acid has shown to decrease bacterial adherence to the epithelial cells lining the urethra, ureters and bladder. (3) Clinically, 60 adults with acute urinary tract infection who consumed 16 ounces of cranberry juice per day showed significant symptomatic improvement within three weeks of treatment. (4) In another study of 22 subjects with UTIs who consumed 15 ounces of cranberry juice per day, 15 showed significant decrease in bacterial adherence as measured by urine clearance collected 3 hours after ingestion of the juice. (3) From these studies it is evident that consumption of large quantities of undiluted cranberry juice is necessary to achieve therapeutic results in treating urinary tract infections.

BOTANICAL MEDICINES

Bearberry (Arctostaphylos uva-ursi) is a low growing evergreen shrub that forms a dark green carpet of leaves. The plant grows abundantly throughout the northern hemisphere in Asia, Europe and northern United States and Canada. Uva-ursi has been used traditionally for centuries as a diuretic, astringent and urinary antiseptic in the treatment of urethritis, cystitis, urinary tract inflammations, kidney stones and bronchitis. (5)

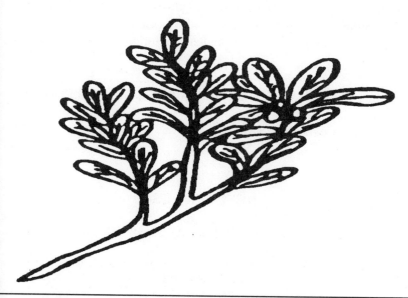

Bearberry (Arctostaphylos uva-ursi)

Uva-ursi contains as it 5 to 18% (usually 7 to 9%) arbutin and methyl arbutin which has been identified as the active ingredient of this plant. The leaves also contain up to 40% tannins responsible for the plant's astringent properties and flavonoids including quercitin. (6)

Arbutin itself is converted by stomach acid in the digestive tract to hydroquinone. Tannins in the plant prevent digestive enzymes from converting arbutin into hydroquinone, which explains why the crude plant is more effective than the pure arbutin extract. (7) In alkaline urine hydroquinone is mildly astringent and is an effective antimicrobial agent. Evidence suggests that arbutin itself may contribute to the antiseptic activity of the plant since both arbutin and the crude leaf extracts have been shown to possess mild antimicrobial activity. Several other compounds in the plant are mild diuretics and contribute to the diuretic effects of the plant. Hydroquinone is rapidly oxidized in alkaline urine which contributes to its antiseptic effects. Uva-ursi is an effective urinary antiseptic. (7)

The ingestion of 1 gram of the compound has resulted in tinnitus (ringing in ears), nausea, vomiting, cyanosis and collapse. Death has resulted following the ingestion of 5 gram of hydroquinone. These side effects are rarely noted because most uva-ursi products deliver less than 1 gram total of uva-ursi. Doses of up to 20 grams of uva-ursi have not caused any side effects in healthy individuals. The astringent tannins of this plant may cause stomach upset and will usually limit the dose when ingested. Uva-ursi use is not recommended during pregnancy. (8)

RECOMMENDATIONS: Daily unless otherwise stated

Cranberry juice (unsweetened)..............................16 ounces (450 grams)
A. uva-ursi (4:1)...750-1500 mg

REFERENCES

(1) Branch WT: Office Practice of Medicine. WB Saunders Company, Philadelphia, Pennsylvania, 1987
(2) The Lawrence Review of Natural Products: Cranberry. Pharmaceutical Information Associates Ltd. Levittown, Pennsylvania, August 1987
(3) Sobota AE: Inhibition of bacterial adherence by cranberry juice: potential use for the treatment of urinary tract infections. J. Urology 131:1013-16, 1984

(4) Papas PN et al: Cranberry juice in the treatment of urinary tract infections. Southwestern Medicine 47:17, 1968

(5) The Lawrence Review of Natural Products: Uva ursi. Pharmaceutical Information Associateds Ltd, Levittown, Pennsylvania, Sept. 1987

(6) Leung A: Encyclopedia of Common Natural Ingredients Used in Food, Drugs, and Cosmetics. John Wiley & Sons, New York, NY, 1980

(7) Frohne V: Untersuchungen zur frage der hamdesifizierenden wirkungen von barentraubenblatt-extracten. Planta Medica 18:1-25, 1970

(8) Merck Index, 10th edition, Merck & Co., Rahway, NJ. 112-13, 1983

CHAPTER 4

CURING CHRONIC YEAST INFECTION

Chronic Yeast Infection is the term used to describe chronic infection of the skin, mouth, digestive system and vagina in females and is a common cause of discomfort and illness. Since the advent of antibiotics in the 1940's the medical establishment has paid little attention to yeast infection. It wasn't until the publication of "The Missing Diagnosis" by O. Truss in 1983 and "The Yeast Connection" by W.G. Crook in 1984 that yeast infection became a legitimate cause of disease and illness. The exact prevalence of Chronic Yeast Infection is not known, but it has been estimated that 20 to 40% of people will experience at least one yeast infection at one point in their life. A significant number of these individuals will experience a second and subsequent yeast infections. Excessive consumption of sugar and refined carbohydrates and long term antibiotic use are the most causes of Chronic Yeast Infection. The medical history is the single most important factor to confirm the diagnosis of yeast infection. A Candida Questionnaire is an important screening questionnaire to help identify those individuals at risk for developing yeast infections

Symptoms of Chronic Yeast Infection include fatigue or lethargy, feeling of being drained, drowsiness, inability to concentrate, feeling of "spaciness" or "unreality", depression, mood swings, headaches, dizziness or loss of balance, pressure above the ears, feeling of head swelling and tingling, recurrent infection or fluids in ears, ear pain or deafness, blurred vision, burning or tearing of eyes, itchy eyes, nasal congestion or discharge, post-nasal drip, itchy nose, dry mouth, rash or blisters in mouth, sore throat, cough, bad breath, pain or tightness in chest, wheezing or shortness of breath, heartburn, indigestion, excessive beltching, abdominal pain, bloating, constipation diarrhea, excessive flatulence, hemorrhoids, rectal itching, painful or burning urination, frequent urination, frequent bladder infections, persistent vaginal itch, persistent vaginal burning, impotence, loss of sexual desire, menstrual cramps and/or other menstrual irregularities, premenstrual tension, muscle aches, muscle weakness and/or paralysis, pain and/or swelling in joints, skin rashes, and increased sensitivities to foods and environmental allergens. (1,2)

Chronic Yeast Infection may be caused by many different factors that lead to Candida overgrowth. Risk factors for Candida overgrowth include the use of anti-ulcer drugs, broad spectrum antibiotics, corticosteroids, oral contraceptives, excessive consumption of sugar, immune deficiency, diabetes mellitus, intravascular catheters, intravenous drug use, lack of digestive enzymes, nutrient deficiency, and prolonged white blood cell deficiency. A high sugar diet and antibiotic use are the most common causes of Candida overgrowth. Sugar is the preferred food source for yeast organisms and a high sugar diet fuels candida overgrowth. Antibiotics are normally given to combat overgrowth by bad bacteria that invade the body and produce infection. Antibiotics kill the good bacteria that normally prevent Candida overgrowth as well as the bad bacteria.

Drug therapy is the focus of conventional medical treatment of Chronic Yeast Infection. Most fungi are resistant to the action of antibacterial drugs and only a few substances have been discovered that exert an inhibitory effect on fungi. Antifungal drugs used by the medical community include Amphotericin B, Flucytosine, Griseofulvin, Nystatin, Clotrimazole, Miconazole, Metronidazole (Flagyl) and Candicidin. Antifungal drugs are relatively toxic and can adversely affect the liver, kidneys, bone marrow and nervous system. Allergic reactions to these drugs can include fever, skin rashes, white blood cell deficiency and serum sickness. Direct toxic reactions to these drugs can include, headache, nausea, vomiting, diarrhea, photosensitivity, anemia, liver damage, kidney damage, bone marrow suppression, electrolyte imbalance, hair loss and mental confusion. While drug therapy may be necessary in some cases of Chronic Yeast Infection, drug therapy should be avoided if possible. Safe and effective natural therapies are available to treat Chronic Yeast Infection. (9)

DIET

The anti-candida diet is designed to eliminate all yeast, fungi, sugar and refined carbohydrates from the diet. Althought it is strict, it is very successful in eliminating Chronic Yeast Infection. The diet must be followed for one to three months for beneficial results. (1,2)

FOOD YOU MUST AVOID

Foods you must avoid include sugar and all refined carbohydrates, all breads and pastries containing yeast, all alcoholic beverages, malt products, condiments, sauces and vinegar containing foods, processed and smoked meats, dried and candied fruits, fruit juices, coffee, tea and other caffeine containing beverages, melons, mushrooms, yeast and other edible fungi, milk, cheese and other dairy products, all vitamin and mineral supplements containing yeast derivatives, some nuts including peanuts and most packaged and processed foods.

Although certain antibiotics are necessary in treating infection, most respiratory infections are caused by viruses and do not respond to antibiotic therapy. Indiscriminate prescription of antibiotics by doctors for viral infections only contributes to Candida overgrowth. Unless necessary, avoid antibiotics including penicillin, streptomycin, ampicillin, amoxicillin, Kefex (R), Ceclor (R), Septra (R) and Bactrim (R).

FOOD YOU CAN EAT

Foods which can be eaten include all vegetables, fresh fruits, lean meats, eggs, certain beverages including herbal teas, whole grains and various nuts, seeds and oils.

NUTRIENTS

Nutrient deficiencies are common in individuals with chronic Candidiasis. Deficiencies of vitamin A, vitamin B2 (riboflavin), vitamin B6 (pyridoxine), folic acid, zinc, selenium, magnesium, iron and essential fatty acids have been observed in individuals with chronic Candidiasis. Supplementation with these vitamins and minerals can improve immune function and prevent Candidal overgrowth. (10,11)

Caprylic acid is a naturally occuring medium chain fatty acid that inhibits the growth of fungi including Candida albicans. Caprylic acid is rapidly absorbed and time release preparations are recommended to allow for slow, uniform release throughout the entire length of the gastrointestinal tract. Caprylic acid is then able to be released in the colon where Candida overgrowth is most prominant. Although the exact mechanism of yeast inhibitory action is not known, caprylic acid is believed to dissolve in the cell membrane of yeast, causing changes in fluidity that lead to membrane disintegration. Caprylic acid may be used with antibiotics and Lactobacillus acidophilus to balance the normal microflora of the body. Caprylic acid is virtually non-toxic and non-sensitizing and should be consumed with meals. It is recommended that any kind of dietary fat such as milk, butter or salad oil be included at meals when caprylic acid is taken. (12,13)

Undecylenic acid is another naturally occuring medium chain fatty acid that inhibits the growth of fungus. Undecylenic acid is particulary effective in treating fungal infections of the skin and is the major ingredient in Desenex (R), a common topical antifungal used to treat foot fungus. Oral preparations containing undecylenic acid may be effective in treating intestinal candidiasis. (12)

Lactobacillus acidophilus is one of a group of naturally occuring bacteria that populate the gastrointestinal tract in humans. Other beneficial lactobacillus species include L. bifidus, L. fermentum, L. casea, L. salivores, L. brevis and L. plantarum. Lactobacillus bacteria are a part of the normal flora of the gastrointestinal tract and do not produce infection or disease. Lactobacillus species are also a part of the normal flora of the vagina in females. Lactobacilli are first introduced into the sterile intestines of the infant through breastfeeding and continue to proliferate until they are a firmly established part of the normal flora. As part of the "normal flora" they inhibit the growth of other bacteria and fungi in both the digestive system and the vagina. They inhibit bacteria and fungi by competition for nutrients, alteration of pH, oxygen utilization, prevention of attachment and production of antibiotic substances. Lactobacilli are capable of producing a number of natural antibiotics that include acidolin, acidophilin, lactocidin, lactobacillin and lactobrevin. In addition, lactobacilli can produce hydrogen peroxide, lactic acid, acetic acid and other inhibitory substances that prevent the growth of bacteria, viruses and fungi. L. acidophilus has consistently shown to retard the growth of Candida albicans. Supplementation with Lactobacillus acidophilus can help repopulate the normal gastrointestinal or vaginal flora and prevent the overgrowth of yeast. (13,14)

Dietary fiber is very important in regulating the health of the digestive system and provides an environment suitable for friendly bacteria. Dietary fiber increases the stool transit time, increases pancreatic secretions, increases bile production, increases production of short chain fatty acids and maintains a healthy bacterial population in the colon. The digestion and fermentation of fiber by the friendly intestinal bacteria results in the production of short chain fatty acids. These short chain fatty acids including acetate, proprionate and butyrate decrease intestinal pH and thereby provides an acidic environment not suitable for other bacteria and fungi. Acetate and proprionate are absorbed by the body and metabolized by the liver to produce energy. Butyrate is the preferred source of energy for intestinal cells and a healthy intestine depends on a high fiber content to provide butyrate. Fiber has a high capacity to bind Candida toxins and antigens and prevent their absorption into the bloodstream. (15,16)

BOTANICAL MEDICINES

Purple coneflower (Echinacea angustifolia) is a perennial flower of the Great Plains of North America that was widely used by the Plain indians. Echinacea contains about 1.0% glycosides known as echinacin that possess immune stimulating activity. Two hundred and three patients with recurrent vaginal candidiasis were treated with antifungal drugs. Those patients also treated with Echinacea extracts experienced significantly lower recurrences of candida infections. It was agreed that Echinacea extracts improved immune response and strengthened the body's ability to fight infection. (17,18)

Garlic (Allium sativum) is a common, strong scented perennial herb native to Europe, central Asia and has been naturalized in North America and is cultivated worldwide. The fresh or dehydrated bulb has been used medicinally for thousands of years. Garlic bulb contains 0.1 to 0.36% volatile oil consisting of allicin and other sulphur containing compounds. Based on various studies, the antimicrobial activity of garlic is due to the sulphur-containing volatile oils. Garlic is a potent broad spectrum antibiotic against various bacteria, viruses and fungi. Garlic's broad spectrum antibiotic activity rivals penicillin. Antifungal effects of garlic have been demonstrated against various Candida species, Trichophyton, Microsporum, Cryptoccocus, Epidermophyton and Histoplasm. Garlic is especially effective against Candida albicans and is more potent than Nystatin, gentian violet and other antifungal drugs. (19,20)

Goldenseal (Hydrastis canadensis) is a small perennial plant growing up to 30 centimeters in height in damp woods and meadows of eastern United States and Canada. Goldenseal has a rough, wrinkled root with a distinctive odor and bitter taste. The Cherokee indians used goldenseal to treat skin ulcers and wounds. Goldenseal root contains 4.0 to 11.0% isoquinoline alkaloids including berberine, berberastine and hydrastine. These alkaloids have demonstrated potent antimicrobial activity against various bacteria, viruses and fungi. Antifungal activity has been demonstrated against Candida, Cryptococcus, Microsporum, Sporothrix and Trichophyton. Berberine is particularly effective against intestinal parasites that cause infectious diarrhea. Berberine is effective against cholera, amebiasis and giardiasis. Berberine also stimulates the immune system by increasing blood supply to the spleen and by activating macrophages, an important white blood cell. Berberine and other related alkaloids are safe and relatively non-toxic. There use during pregnancy is not recommended. (21,22)

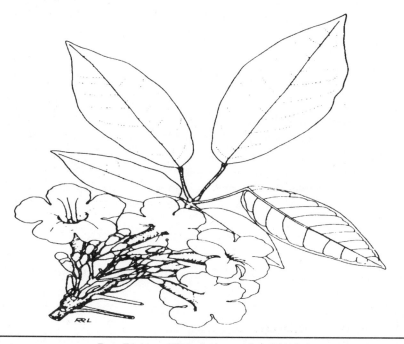

Pau D' Arco (Tabebuia avellanedae)

Pau D' Arco (Tabebuia avellanedae) also known as LaPacho or Taheebo, is a tree native to South America that can grow to a height of 125 feet. Pau D' Arco has become extremely popular as a folk remedy to treat intestinal and vaginal yeast infections. The inner bark and heartwood has been used by South American indians to treat a variety of afflictions including infections and cancer. The heartwood of Pau D' Arco contains 2.0 to 7.0% quinone derivatives primarily as lapachol. These quinone derivatives are responsible for antimicrobial activity of this plant. Antifungal activity has been demonstrated against Candida albicans and Trichophyton. Pau D' Arco is relatively non-toxic, but chronic use can lead to anemia. The usual form of administration of Pau D' Arco is a tea and the standard dose is usually two to eight cups of tea per day. (23,24)

Australian tea tree (Melaleuca alternifolia) is a small tree native only to the northeast region of Australia. The leaves of this plant contain about 1.0 to 3.0% of an oil that has demonstrated significant antiseptic and antifungal activity. Antifungal activity of tea tree oil has been demonstrated against Candida albicans and Trichophyton. Tea tree preparations have been used successfully to treat athlete's foot, ringworm, jock itch, skin and vaginal infections, tinea, thrush and bacterial infection. Topical tea tree preparations are safe and non-toxic. A tea made from boiling the leaves of this plant is also safe. However, the oil is toxic when taken internally and oral consumption of the oil is not recommended. (25,26)

Many other botanical medicines contain essential oils that demonstrate significant antifungal activity. Peppermint (Mentha piperita), Ginger (Zingiber officinale), Chamomile (Matricaria chamomilla), Thyme (Thymus vulgaris), Balm (Melissa officinale), Rosemary (Rosmarinus officinalis), Cinnamon (Cinnamomum verum). Liberal consumption of these herbs is recommended as teas or spices. (27,28)

RECOMMENDATIONS: Daily unless otherwise stated

Vitamin A..10,000-20,000 IU
Vitamin B2 (Riboflavin)..10-25 mg
Vitamin B6 (Pyridoxine)...25-50 mg
Folic Acid..200-400 mcg

Iron...10-25 mg
Magnesium...400-800 mg
Selenium...200-400 mcg
Zinc...25-50 mg
Essential Fatty Acids..3-6 gm
Caprylic Acid...1-2 gm
Undecylenic Acid..1-2 gm
Lactobacillus acidophilus....................................1-3 tsp
Dietary Fiber...20-40 gm
Echinacea angustifolia (6.5:1)...........................500-1000 mg
Allium sativum (Fresh Garlic)............................10-20 gm
Hydrastis canadensis (4:1)...............................500-1000 mg
Pau D' Arco (Taheebo)(4:1)..............................2 to 8 cups of tea
Tea Tree Oil...................................Apply topically as directed

REFERENCES

(1) Crook WA: The Yeast Connection: A Medical Breakthrough. Professional Books, Jackson, Tennesee, 1984.

(2) Truss O: The Missing Diagnosis. P.O. Box 26508, Birmingham, Alabama, 1983

(3) Pizzorno JE and Murray MT: Textbook of Natural Medicine. JBC Publications, Seattle, Washington, 1988.

(4) Kroker GF: Chronic candidiasis and allergy. In: Brostoff J and Challacombe SJ (eds): Food Allergy and Intolerance. WB Saunders, Philadelphia, Penn., pp. 850-72, 1987.

(5) Boero M et al: Candida overgrowth in gastric juice of peptic ulcer subjects on short- and long-term treatment with H2-receptor antagonists. Digestion 28:153-63, 1983

(6) Rubinstein E et al: Antibacterial activity of the pancreatic fluid. Gastroenterol. 88:927-32, 1985

(7) Technical Support. Vol. 1 No. 3 and No. 4: Vaginal Mycosis (Part I and II), Probiologic Inc., Bellevue, Washington, October, 1987 and February, 1988.

(8) Abe F et al: Experimental candidiasis in liver injury. Mycopathogia 100:37-42, 1987

(9) Berkow R (ed): The Merck Manual of Diagnosis and Therapy (15th ed.) Merck, Sharp & Dohme Laboratories, Rahway, N.J. 1987

(10) Galland L: Nutrition and candidiasis. J. Orthomol. Psychiatry 15:50-60, 1986.(11) Hoffman C et al: Fungistatic Properties of Fatty Acids and Possible Biochemical Significance. Food Research 4:539, 1939

(12) Tsukahara T: Fungicidal Action of Caprylic Acid for Candida albicans. Japan J. Microbiology. Vol. 5 No. 4, 1961

(13) Collins EB et al: Inhibition of Candida albicans by Lactobacillus acidophilus. J. Dairy Sci. 63:830-2, 1980

(14) Shani KM et al: Role of Natural Antibiotic activity of Lactobacillus acidophilus and bulgaricus. Cult. Dairy Prod. J. 12:8-11, 1977

(15) Anderson JW et al: Plant fiber: Carbohydrate and Lipid Metabolism. The American

J. of Clin. Nutr. 32:346-63, February, 1979
(16) Vahouny G et al: Dietary Fiber in Health and Disease. Plenum Press, New York, NY, 1982.
(17) Kindscher K: Ethnobotany of Purple coneflower (Echinacea angustifolia, Asteraceae) and other Echinacea species. Ethnobotany 43(4):498-507, 1989
(18) Coeugniet E et al: Recurrent candidiasis: Adjuvant immunotherapy with different formulations of Echinacin. Therapiewocke 36 p. 3352-58, Heft 33, August 1986.(19) Adetumbi MA et al: Allium sativum (garlic) - A natural antibiotic. Med. Hypothesis 12:227-37, 1983
(20) Moore GS et al: The fungicidal and fungistatic effects of an aqueous garlic extract on medically important yeast-like fungi. Mycologia 69:341-8, 1977
(21) Hahn FE et al: Berberine. Antibiotics 3:577-88, 1976
(22) Mahajan VM et al: Antimycotic activity of berberine sulphate: An alklaoid from an Indian medicinal herb. Sabouraudia 20:79-81, 1982
(23) Willard T: Tabebuia Species: In: A Textbook of Natural Medicine. Pizzorno JE and Murray MT (eds). JBC Publications, Seattle, WA. pp. Chapter V: Tabebuia, 1987
(24) The Lawrence Review of Natural Products: Taheebo. Lawrence Review. Collegeville, Penn. May 1986
(25) Altman PM: Australian Tea Tree Oil. Current Drug Information. Vol. 2, pp. 62-4, April 1988
(26) Essential Oils Data Search Inc: Melaleuca alternifolia, a compilation of articles and papar about Australian tea tree oil. Vancouver, WA, 1985
(27) Duke JA: Handbook of Medicinal Herbs. CRC Press. Boca Raton, FL., 1985
(28) Leung AYL Encyclopedia of Common Natural Ingredients Used in Food, Drugs, and Cosmetics. John Wiley & Sons, New York, NY., 1980

CHAPTER 5

DECREASING HIGH BLOOD PRESSURE

Hypertension or high blood pressure is defined as a blood pressure greater than 140/90. Hypertension is a disease of modern society and is estimated to affect 20 to 40% of the North American population. Direct consequences of hypertension resulting from the increased blood pressure include congestive heart failure, aneurysm, cerebral hemorrhage and blood vessel rupture. Indirect consequences of hypertension resulting from decreased blood flow and lack of oxygen include heart attack, kidney sclerosis (hardening)) and stroke. Atherosclerosis, hardening of the arteries, contributes to elevated blood pressure by increasing vascular resistance. Risk factors that contribute to an elevation of blood pressure include hyperlipidemia (high fat level in circulating blood), diabetes mellitus, cigarette smoking, atherosclerosis and advanced age. Current evidence suggests that genetic factors may increase the predisposition to high blood pressure. Essential hypertension is estimated to affect 90 to 95% of all hypertensives and has no known cause. Safe and natural alternatives are available for the treatment of high blood pressure.

DIET

A high fiber diet is associated with decrease in blood pressure. (1) A low fat diet with a high percentage of polyunsaturated fats (PUFAs) and low saturated fats lowers blood pressure. (2) Refined carbohydrates, especially sugar and excess alcohol consumption raises blood pressure. (3,4) An increased consumption of raw, uncooked foods has a corresponding lowering effect on blood pressure. (5) Caffeine intake has a direct immediate effect in raising blood pressure and should be eliminated from the diet. (6) A vegetarian diet high in fiber, vegetable protein, unsaturated fats, potassium and magnesium results in a significant decrease in blood pressure. (7)

NUTRIENTS

A decrease in Vitamin A intake was associated with an increase in blood pressure. (8)

Vitamin B complex supplementation in association with dietary factors has demonstrated to be very beneficial in lowering blood pressure in hypertensives. (9)

A lower intake of ascorbic acid (Vitamin C) has been correlated with elevated blood pressure. (8)

Vitamin D supplementation may be beneficial in lowering blood pressure. (10)

Reduced dietary calcium intake is significantly associated with the development of high blood pressure. It has been postulated that abnormal calcium homeostasis may be a primary factor in the development of hypertension. The association of low dietary calcium with increased development of hypertension is greater than high sodium intake and the development of blood pressure. Supplementation with calcium results in a significant decrease in blood pressure levels. (11)

Magnesium is a potent vasodilator because of its ability to displace calcium from vascular smooth muscle. (12) A significant decrease in potassium intake is associated with high blood pressure. (8)

Sodium restriction may delay or prevent the development of hypertension. Sodium restriction to 2 grams per day has been shown to be manageable and safe and probably will benefit hypertensive patients who are sodium sensitive. (4)

Supplementation with coenzyme Q10 which is often deficient in hypertensives, results in a significant decrease in blood pressure. (13)

Essential fatty acids supplementation as omega-3 and omega-6 oils also is beneficial in lowering blood pressure. (14)

OTHER FACTORS

Food sensitivities have been implicated in the development of high blood pressure. An elimination diet results in elimination of the suspected food allergy and results in a decrease in blood pressure. (17)

Cadmium and lead toxicities have been suspected to affect blood pressure levels. (18) Zinc supplementation appears to reverse cadmium associated hypertension. (19)

BOTANICAL MEDICINES

Garlic (Allium sativa) is a strong scented perennial herb with long, flat and firm leaves, widely used as a culinary spice in cooking. Garlic has been used medicinally for thousands of years by various cultures in the treatment of colds, respiratory infections, whooping cough, bronchitis, toothache, earache and many other conditions too numerous to list.

Garlic contains 0.1 to 0.36% volatile oil composed of allicin, allylpropyl disulfide, diallyl disulfide and diallyl trisulfide as the major components. (15) The volatile oil component of garlic is responsible for this plant's unmistakable pungent odor. Allicin, the major odor principle, is produced by the enzymatic action of allinase on allin, a non-volatile component, by the crushing of the bulb.

Garlic and garlic oil have numerous pharmacologic activities including antimicrobial activity; antibacterial, antiviral, antifungal and antihelmintic effects, anti-atherosclerotic effects, hypocholesterolemic effects, platelet aggregation inhibition, fibrinolytic effects, antitumor effects and anti-inflammatory effects. (16)

Garlic also has hypotensive effects and should be consumed liberally to lower elevated blood pressure. Clinical investigation of raw garlic on 21 hypertensive patients and an extract prepared from garlic leaves on 46 hypertensive patients showed a moderate hypotensive effect. Systolic pressure dropped by 20 to 30 mm Hg and the diastolic pressure dropped 10 to 20 mm Hg. (Note: mm Hg stands for millimeters of mercury and are standard units of blood pressure measurement.) (17) Other clinical investigations with animal and human models has consistently demonstrated significant hypotensive action. (18) Garlic is a versatile plant with many different medicinal effects and marked hypotensive effects. Garlic should be consumed daily to lower high blood pressure. Ten to thirty grams of fresh garlic or the equivalent dose of a standardized garlic preparation is the recommended dose.

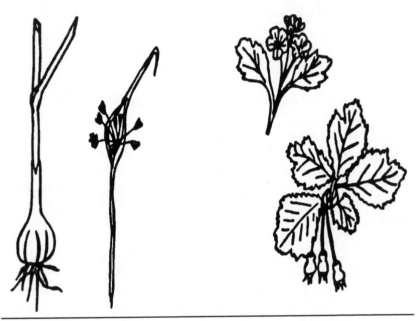

Garlic (Allium sativum)   Hawthorn (Crataegus oxyacantha)

Hawthorn (Crataegus oxyacantha), a member of the Rose family, is a tree or shrub that grows throughout Europe, east Asia and eastern North America. Crataegus contains over 30 different flavonoids ranging from 0.05 to 5.0% total flavonoid content. The flavonoids are a group of naturally occurring compounds that are responsible, in part, for the color of the fruits of hawthorn and other members of the Rose family.

Active flavonoids in hawthorn include proanthocyanidins, anthocyanidins, rutin, catechin and flavone derivatives such as hyperoside and vitexin-4'-rhamnoside. (19) The flavonoids in Crataegus are responsible for this plant's ability to increase blood flow to the heart, increase the contractile force of heart contraction, decrease oxygen use by the heart muscle and decrease blood pressure. The hypotensive effects of Crataegus are indirect and due to its ability to improve heart function. The hypotensive action of Crataegus, although significant, is of short duration and its use in controlling high blood pressure should be supplemented with other botanical medicines. (17)

European mistletoe (Viscum album) is a parasitic, woody perennial commonly found growing on oaks and other deciduous trees throughout Europe. Early pagan custom required hanging mistletoe over doors and in hallways to inspire passion in the pagan holiday, "Hoeul". Today, these evergreen plants are used as a Christmas ornament and the custom of kissing under the plant is a keyed-down version of this ancient pagan practice. (20)

The chemical constituents of mistletoe reflects the chemical constituents of the host plant on which this parasite grows. Mistletoe contains alkaloids, vaso-active amines, sterols, flavonoids, toxic proteins designated viscotoxins and a toxic lectin called viscumin. (21)

The pharmacologic effects of European mistletoe on the the cardiovascular system include vasodilating action, cardiac depressant and hypotensive actions. (17) The exact chemical constituents responsible for these effects have not been clearly identified and it has been proposed that various constituents exert a combined synergisitic action. Viscum extracts appear to act on the vasomotor centre regulating blood pressure control in the medulla oblongata in the brain. Viscum has also demonstrated cholinomimetic activity that may activate the parasympathetic nervous system and cause vasodilation. Aqueous extracts of Viscum contain proteins and lectins that have shown significant hypotensive effects. In Europe, over 150 different proprietary medicines contain mistletoe and mistletoe extracts and a number of these medicines are specific for treatment of hypertension. (22)

Mistletoe is a toxic plant and should only be administered under medical supervision. Symptoms of toxicity include allergic reactions, nausea, slow heart rate, gastroenteritis, diarrhea and vomiting. Overdose of mistletoe has resulted in death. Under proper medical supervision mistletoe is safe and effective in treating hypertension. Use of this plant during pregnancy is not recommended. (23)

Ginkgo biloba, is one of the world's oldest living trees and its history can be traced back more than 200 million years. Ginkgo contains a high content of flavonoids, proanthocyanidins, terpenes and flavonolignans termed Ginkgo heterosides. Standardized Ginkgo biloba extracts contain 24% ginkgo heterosides. Ginkgo causes peripheral dilation in blood vessels and has been used to treat transient ischemic attacks, stroke, headache, tinnitus, macular degeneration in the eye, diabetic retinopathy and intermittent claudication. Ginkgo inhibits platelet aggregation, stabilizes cellular membranes, decreases membrane permeability, stimulates the synthesis of prostanoids and related substances that dilate blood vessels and has demonstrated potent antioxidant action. (24)

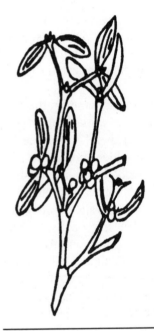
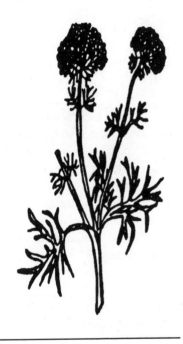

Mistletoe (Viscum album)   Khella (Ammi visnaga)

     Khella (Ammi visnaga) is a plant native to the Mediterranean and Egypt and was used for thousands of years since the time of the pharoahs. Khella contains lactone glycosides mainly as coumarin and furanocoumarins which inhibit cAMP phosphodiesterase, the enzyme responsible conversion of cAMP to cGMP. The net effect of increased cAMP levels is relaxation of smooth muscle around vessels resulting in vasodilation. Khella has been used in the treatment of cardiovascular disease and hypertension. (25)

RECOMMENDATIONS: Daily unless otherwise stated

Vitamin A	10,000-50,000 IU
Vitamin B-complex	50-100 mg
Vitamin C	1000-5000 mg
Vitamin D	400 IU
Calcium	1000-2000 mg
Magnesium	400-800 mg
Zinc	25 mg
Coenzyme Q10	60 mg
Omega-3 oil (Max EPA)	5-10 gm
Omega-6 oil (Evening primrose oil)	5-10 gm
Allium sativum (Fresh garlic)	1-3 gm
Crataegus oxyacantha (4:1)	1000-2000 mg
Viscum album (5:1)	100-200 mg
Ginkgo biloba (8:1)	120-240 mg
Ammi visnaga (10:1)	300-600 mg

REFERENCES

(1) Burr ML et al: Dietary fibre, blood pressure and plasma cholesterol. Nutr. Res. 5:465-72,. 1985

(2) Iacono JM et al: Reduction of blood pressure associated with dietary polyunsaturated fat. Hypertension 4(suppl III):III-34, 1982

(3) Aherns RA: Fed. Proc. vol. 34, 1975

(4) Non-pharmacologic approaches to the control of high blood pressure. Final report of the subcommittee on non-pharmacologic therapy of the 1984 Joint National Committe on Detection, Evaluation and Treatment of High Blood Pressure. Hypertension 8(5):444-67, 1986

(5) Douglass J et al: Effects of a raw food diet on hypertension and obesity. South. Med. J. 78(7):841, 1985

(6) Smith P et al: Circulatory effects of coffee in relation to the pharmacokinetics of caffeine. Am. J. Cardiology 56(15):958-63, 1985

(7) Rouse IL et al: Blood pressure lowering effects of a vegetarian diet. Lancet 1:5-9. 1983

(8) McCarron DA et al: Blood pressure and nutrient intake in the United States. Science 224(4656):1392-8, 1984

(9) Vodoevich VP et al: Effect of the B-group vitamin complex on the blood content of saturated and unsaturated fatty acids in patients with ischemic heart disease and hypertension. Vopr. Pitan. (2):9-11, 1986

(10) Sowers MF et al: The association of intakes of vitamin D and blood among women. Am. J. Clin. Nutr. 42:135-42, 1985

(11) McCarron DA: Is calcium more important than sodium in the pathogenesis of essential hypertension? Hypertension 7(4):607-27, 1985

(12) Altura BT: Interactions of Mg and K on blood vessels: Aspects in view of hypertension. Magnesium 3(3-6):175-94, 1984

(13) Yamagami T et al: Correlation between serum Q levels and succinate dehydrogenase coenzyme Q reductase activity in cardiovascular disease and the influence of coenzyme Q administration. Biomed. & Clin. Aspects of Coenzyme Q. Science Publishers, Amsterdam, Elsevier, pp. 253-62, 1984

(14) Norris PG et al: Effect of dietary supplementation with fish oil on systolic blood pressure in mild hypertension. Br. Med. J. 293:104, 1986

(15) Leung AY: Encylcopedia of Common Natural Ingredients Used in Food, Drugs, and Cosmetics. John Wiley & Sons, New York, NY, 1980

(16) Block E: The Chemistry of Garlic and Onions. Scientific American. pp. 114-119, March 1985

(17) Petkov V: Plants with Hypotensive, Antiatheromatous and Coronarodilating Action. Am. J. of Chinese Med. Vol. VII No. 7, pp. 197-236, 1979

(18) Lau B et al: Allium sativum (Garlic) and Atherosclerosis: A review. Nutrition Research Vol. 3, pp. 1190128, 1983

(19) Ammon HPT et al: Crataegus, Toxikologie und Pharmakologie Teil II: Pharmakodynamik. Planta Medica Vol. 43 No. 3, November 1981

(20) Becker H: Botany of European Mistletoe (Viscum album L.). Oncology 43(suppl. 1):2-7, 1986

(21) Wagner H et al: Studies on the standardization of mistletoe preparations. Oncology 43(suppl. 1):8-15, 1896

(22) Anderson LA et al: Mistletoe - the magic herb

(23) Duke JA: Handbook of Medicinal Herbs. CRC Press, Boca Raton, FL. pp. 512-3, 1986

(24) Vorberg G: Gingko biloba extract (GBE): A long term study of chronic cerebral vascular insufficiency in geriatric patients. Clin. Trials. J. 22:149-57, 1985

(25) Thastrup O et al: Coronary vasodilating, spasmolytic and cAMP phosphodiesterase inhibitory properties of dihydropyranocoumarins and dihydrofuranocoumarins. Acta Pharmac. et. Toxicol. 52:246-53, 1983

CHAPTER 6

ELIMINATING ANXIETY AND STRESS

Anxiety is defined as an unusual state of arousal or excitment. Anxiety is punctuated by mental uneasiness, worry, a sense of doom or impending terror. Anxiety can manifest as outright panic attacks. Other forms of anxiety include post-traumatic stress disorder, obsessive compulsive disorder, somatoform disorder, bipolar disorder and depression. Approximately 10% of the entire population experiences anxiety. It is estimated that 50 to 70% of patient visits to doctors have some anxiety or stress-related component. Physical symptoms of anxiety include insomnia, heart palpitations, missed or skipped heart beats, rapid heart beat, fast, shallow breathing, sweating, trembling, queasiness or upset stomach, diarrhea, gas, bloating, muscle weakness and fatigue.. It is important to mention that many other diseases can cause anxiety including thyroid disease, lung disorders, hormone disorders and heart attacks.

The exact cause of anxiety is not known. Higher circulating levels of adrenal hormones such as adrenaline have been associated with higher levels of arousal, anxiety and panic attacks. Higher levels of lactate have also been associated with chronic anxiety. Lactate is a metabolic product of sugar breakdown in the body. Under normal circumstances glucose is broken down slowly in the presence of oxygen. Under stressful conditions glucose is broken down quickly without oxygen. The end product of the anaerobic breakdown of glucose is lactate. Intravenous injections of lactate produced high levels of anxiety and panic attacks.

The standard medical treatment for anxiety is drug therapy. Commonly prescribed medication include, anti-anxiety drugs, anti-depressants and tranquilizers. The most commonly prescribed medication for anxiety is a group of drugs collectively known as benzodiazepines. These benzodiazepines include such popular drugs as Valium, Librium, Xanax, Serax, Ativan, Restoril and Halcion. In the early 1980's Valium was the most commonly prescribed drug in North America. All these drugs work by potentiating the effect of a brain hormone known as GABA. These drugs are highly addictive, have numerous side effects and are meant for short term use only. There are very effective and safe natural therapies for anxiety and stress

PSYCHOLOGY

Counselling may be effective in helping a person identify specific causes and triggers of anxiety. Stress reduction techniques such as deep breathing, meditation, progressive relaxation, autogenic training, quieting and hypnosis are effective in quelling anxiety and promoting relaxation. Most of these methods are inexpensive, easy to do to do and portable. They must be practiced daily to be effective.

DIET

Avoid alcohol consumption. Alcohol can increase the lactate to pyruvate ratio.(1) Avoid caffeine foods and beverages including coffee, tea, soft drinks and chocolate. Caffeine can increase the lactate to pyruvate ration. (2) Many individuals with anxiety may be unusually sensitive to caffeine. (3) Avoid sugar and sugar containing foods and beverages. Many individuals with anxiety may be unusually sensitive to sugar and sugar products. Sugar stimulates the production of insulin which can lead to a decrease in blood sugar levels. Many individuals with anxiety respond to a hypoglycemic diet. (4) This diet strictly avoids sugar, sweets, caffeine and refined foods. It promotes frequent snacking of protein-rich foods which helps to stabilize blood sugar levels.

NUTRIENTS

Rule out B vitamin deficiency. Vitamin B supplementation helps to support the nervous system. (5) Vitamin B1 supplementation helps to decrease the conversion of pyruvate to lactate. (5) Vitamin B3 supplementation in the form of niacinamide increase the conversion of lactate to pyruvate. (6) Niacinamide has shown to have anti-anxiety, muscle relaxant and hypnotic action comparable to the effectiveness of minor tranquilizers. (7) Vitamin B6 supplementation helps to facilitate the conversion of lactate to pyruvate. (8)

Calcium supplementation has anti-anxiety, muscle relaxant and nerve depressant action. (9) Magnesium deficiency increases the conversion of pyruvate to lactate. Magnesium supplementation has anti-anxiety and muscle relaxant action. (10)

GABA supplementation helps to reduce anxiety, control panic attacks and promote relaxation. GABA, gamma amino butyric acid, is a non-essential amino acid that is utilized in the brain and nervous system. There are specific GABA receptors on nerve cells that inhibit excitation in the nervous system. Benzodiazepine drugs, such as Ativan, Serax, Xanax and Valium work by potentiating the effect of GABA and the GABA receptor. (12) However, these drugs are highly addictive and have many unpleasant side effects. Supplementation with GABA promotes relaxation and quells anxiety. GABA is safe, effective and has very minimal side effects. It can be taken for prolonged periods without risk of addiction. (13)

Supplementation with the amino acid L-Tryptophan decrease anxiety levels. (11) Tryptophan is a precursor to the brain hormone serotonin. Tryptophan and serotonin have a calming, mood elevating and sleep producing effect. (12)

BOTANICAL MEDICINE

Kava kava (Piper methysticum) is a member of the pepper family native to the polynesian islands of the south pacific. The root of the plant has been used medicinally by the indigenous natives of the south pacific for hundreds of years. Kava root has been used for a variety of complaints including pain relief, muscle relaxation, sleep, coughs, colds, infections, headache and fatigue. A ceremonial drink prepared from chewing kava root, mixing it with saliva, water and coconut milk has been incorporated in religious and social occasions. Kava juice is poured in a coconut bowl, passed around a close circle and shared by all. Upon consumption of the juice a person would say "maca" meaning it is empty. The bowl would be refilled and continued to be passed around the circle. Kava would have a mildly intoxicating effect. A person would become happy, relaxed and invigorated. Unlike alcohol or other medication a person's mental faculties would be unaffected.   There would be no morning hangover from kava consumption from the previous night.   Kava was first introduced to westerners during the voyages of Captain James Cook as visited the various islands of the south Pacific. (14)

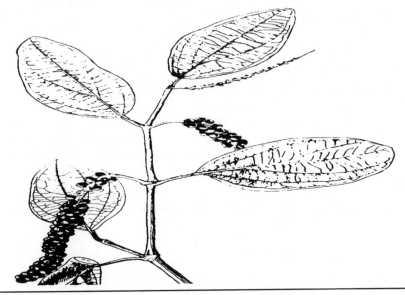

Kava kava (Piper methysticum)

The active ingredients in kava kava are a group of resinous compounds called kavalactones.   The kavalactone content of the root can vary from 3.0 to 20.0%.   Kavalactone resins are found in the fatty portion of the kava root.   High quality herbal extracts are standardized to contain 30% kavalactone content. (15)

Kavalactones have analgesic, anaesthetic, anti-anxiety, anti-convulsant, muscle relaxant and spasmolytic activity. Kavalactones are believed to modulate the GABA receptor in specific parts of the brain and nervous system without actually binding to the receptor itself. GABA is believed to act in a part of the brain called the limbic system which is the main area that affects our emotional responses. Kavalactones are believed to promote muscle relaxation and sedation primarily through it's effect on the limbic system. (15)

Numerous clinical studies confirm the anti-anxiety, muscle relaxant and mood enhancing effects of kava kava. In one double blind study kavalactone extraxt was compared to oxazepam, an anti-anxiety drug similar to valium. Over a four week period kava was as effective as oxazepam. It did not alter mental function and their was no dependence. (16) In another clinical study of 84 patients with chronic anxiety were treated with 400 mg of a purified kavalactone extract. Kava was shown to decrease all symptoms of anxiety and improved mental function. (17) In another double blind study of 40 menopausal women, kava extract decreased anxiety levels and improved other menopausal symptoms. No side effect were noted. (18) In yet another study, 58 chronic anxiety patients were assigned to one group that took kavalactone extract or the other group took placebo. The group that took kava extract should significant improvement of all symptoms associated with anxiety including nervousness, chest pains, heart palpitations, headache, dizziness and stomach upset. Again no adverse side effects were noted. (19) In another study, of twelve healthy volunteers, kavalactone extract was compared to the anti-anxiety drug oxazepam. While oxazepam caused significant impairment of memory and reaction time, kava showed a slight increased improvement in memory and reaction time. (20)

The dosage of kava kava should reflect kavalactone content. Based on clinical studies the dosage of kavalactone for anxiety control 45 to 90 milligrams three times per day. This translates to a dose of 150 to 300 milligrams of a kava extract standardized to contain 30% kavalactone content. For sleep to sedative effects the dosage can be increased moderately. (15)

Kava kava a low level of toxicity. Occasional allergic reaction, indigestion and stomach upset have been reported. An unusual condition called kava dermotherapy has been reported by a few individuals who consumed larger amounts of kava for prolonged periods of time. The skin can become unusually dry, scaly and flaky, especially on the hands, arms, feet and legs. This condition reverses after kava is discontinued. Very large doses of kava certain blood parameters incuding protein, urea, bilirubin and certain cell counts. Large doses of kava are not recommended. It's use during pregnancy is discouraged. (15)

RECOMMENDATIONS: Daily unless otherwise stated

Vitamin B-complex...50 mg

Vitamin B1...10-25 mg
Vitamin B3..100-500 mg
Vitamin B6...25-50 mg
Calcium...750-1500 mg
Magnesium...500-1000 mg
L-Tryptophan..500-1000 mg
GABA...500-2000 mg
Kava kava (4:1)...150-600 mg

REFERENCES

(1) Albeti KG and Nattrass M: Lancet 2:25-29, 1977

(2) Charney DS et al: Increased anxiogenic effects of caffeine in panic disorder. Arch Gen. Psychiatr. 42:2330243, 1985

(3) Greden JF: Anxiety or caffeinism. A diagnostic dilemma. Am. J.Psychiatr.,Oct. 1974

(4) Rainey JM et al: Psychopharmac. Bull. 20(1)45-9, 1984.

(5) Abbey LC: Agorophophobia. J. Orthomol. Psychiat. 11:243-259, 1982

(6) Mohler H et al: Nicotinamide is a brain consitituen with benzodiazepine-like actions. Nature 278:563-65, 1979

(7) Buist RA: Anxiety neurosis. The lactate connection. Int Clin. Nutr. Rev. 5:1-4, 1985

(8) Buist -RA op cit.

(9) Carlson RJ: Longitudinal oberservations of two case of organice anxiety syndrome. Psychosomatics, 27(7):529-31, 1986

(10) Buist RA op cit.

(11) Hoes M et al: Hyperventilation syndrome, Treatment with L-tryptophan and pyridoxine. J. Orthomol. Psychiat. 10(1):7-15, 1981

(12) Werbach MR: Nutritional Influences on Mental Illness. Third Line Press, Tarzana, CA., 1991

(13) Braverman E and Pfeiffer C: The Healing Nutrients Within: Facts, Findings and New Research on Amino Acids. Keats Publishing, New Canaan, CT, 1987

(14) Lebot V et al: Kava: The Pacific Drug. Yale University Press, New Haven, CT., 1992

(15) Meyer HJ: Pharmacology of Kava: Ethnopharmacological Search for Psychoactive Drugs. Raven Press, New York, NY, pp. 133-40, 1979

(16) Lindenberg D and Pitule-Shodel H: D,L-kavain in comparison to oxazepam in anxiety disorder. Forschr. Med. 108:49-54, 1990

(17) Scholing WE and Clausen HD: On the effect of d,l-kavain: experience with neuronika. Med. Lkin. 72: 1301-6. 1977

(18) Warnecke G: Neurovegetative dystonia in the female climacteric. Fortschr. Med. 109:120-2, 1991

(19) Kinzler E et al: Clinical efficacy of a kava extract in patients with anxiety syndrome. Arzneim. Forsch. 41:585-8, 1991

(20) Munte TF et al: Effects of oxazepam an extract of kava root on event related potentials. Neuropsychobiol. 27:46-53, 1993

CHAPTER 7

ENHANCING BRAIN AND MEMORY

Alzheimer's`s disease (AD) has been called "the disease of the century". Alzheimer's disease is now thought to be the fourth leading cause of death in developed nations, after heart disease, cancer and stroke. Alzheimer's disease is estimated to affect 5 to 10% of the population over the age of 65 and up to 20% of the population over age 80. One of the most feared and devastating aspects of aging is the deterioration of memory and other mental processes that occurs with increasing frequency in advancing years. In 1900 only 4% of the population in Canada and the United States had attained 65 years of age. By 1990, 11% of the population had been estimated to be 65 years or older. The fastest growing segment of today's population in North America is the 80 years and older group. Current demographic projections indicate that this trend will continue and the percentage of individuals 65 years old and older will increase throughout the remainder of this century and afterward as well.

The cause of Alzheimer's disease is unknown. The variety of theories suggests that Alzheimer's disease is multifactorial in origin. Leading theories of the causes of Alzheimer's Disease include: Neurotransmitter or other brain chemical deficits or imbalances (particularly acetylcholine and proteins). Specifically a deficiency of an enzyme called LCAT (lecithin choline acetyltransferase) in certain key parts of the brain has been discovered in ALzheimer's patients. Selective brain cell death or injury induced by viral or other transmissible disease agents in the environment. Excessive accumulation in the brain of aluminum or other toxins. Genetic factors (Defects or predispositions) An autoimmune process (i.e. anti-brain antibodies related to aging). Various nutrient deficiencies are associated with the development of Alzheimer's disease and should be identified and treated accordingly. Treatment should also consist of developing ways of effectively supporting the families of patients with this disease.

DIET

A well balanced diet emphasizing whole, unprocessed and unrefined foods is recommended. Refined carbohydrates, sugar, fat and alcohol should be decreased. Complex carbohydrates, fruit and vegetables and fiber should be increased. Diet should also be rich in choline containing foods such as wheat germ and other complex carbohydrates, nuts, legumes and meat. The diet should include a wide variety of foods to maintain proper nutrition and prevent nutritional deficiencies. (3)

VITAMINS AND MINERALS

Individuals with dementia are more likely to be deficient of various vitamins and minerals than are members of their cohort. (2)

Folic acid deficiency is associated with organic brain syndrome and dementia. Deficiency is associated with apathy, disorientation, poor concentration and memory deficits. (2) Deficiency is common among elderly psychiatric patients and supplementation may be beneficial. (3)

Vitamin B1 (Thiamine) is often deficient in elderly patients suffering from Alzheimer's disease and supplementation may be beneficial is slowing progression of mental deterioration. (4)

Vitamin B6 (Pyridoxine) is often deficient in elderly patients suffering from Alzheimer's disease and parallels an age-related decline in dopamine receptors. (5)

Vitamin B12 deficiency is associated with depression, confusion, memory deficits and mental slowness, along with neurologic deficits. (6) Vitamin B12 levels were significantly lower and deficiency was more frequent in individuals with Alzheimer's dementia. (7) Vitamin B12 supplementation may be effective in improving the symptoms associated with this deficiency.

Vitamin C deficiency is not uncommon among elderly psychiatric patients and deficiency is marked among individuals with senile dementia. (5)

Vitamin E is often deficient in Alzheimer's patients. (8) Individuals with Down's syndrome, who are prone to neurologic degeneration and are at high risk of developing dementia, have increased superoxide dismutase (SOD), which may damage cell membranes because of increased free radicals. (9) Since vitamin E is a free radical scavenger, supplementation may reduce the damage associated cell membrane damage.

The role of aluminum and silicon in the development of Alzheimer's disease is still controversial. Elevated aluminum and silicon levels have been found in brains of patients with Alzheimer dementia. Aluminum has been found to inhibit choline transport in nerve endings, reduces choline acetyltransferase (CAT) activity and is associated with the development of neurofibrillary tangles. (10) It is believed that elevated brain aluminum levels in Alzheimer's dementia may contribute to the neurologic degeneration associated with this disease. If this is the case, then it is advised that aluminum exposure is kept to a minimum.

Excess copper accumulation is known to cause mental deterioration and brain injury. (11)

Excess iron accumulation in brain tissue can act as a pro-oxidant and accelerate free radical damage and brain injury. (12)

Chronically excessive exposure of manganese is associated with an increased risk of dementia. (13)

Most of the enzymes primarily concerned with DNA replication, repair and growth are zinc dependent. Zinc may be deficient in individuals with Alzheimer's disease and administration of zinc could prevent or delay the onset of dementia in subjects genetically at risk. (14)

NUTRIENTS

Lecithin (Phosphatidyl choline) is required for the formation of the neurotransmitter, acetylcholine. (15) Alzheimer's disease is marked by decreased levels of choline acetyltransferase (CAT), the enzyme required for production of acetylcholine. It is logical to assume that supplying the precursors necessary for acetylcholine synthesis would improve Alzheimer's disease. The use of lecithin in treating Alzheimer's disease is still controversial. Lecithin supplementation does not appear to improve the symptoms associated with Alzheimer's disease, but rather appears to useful in retarding the rate of disease progression. (16) The percentage of phosphatidyl choline varies between 10 to 95% in commercially available "phosphatidyl choline" and "lecithin".

Phosphatidylserine is a major phospholipid found in brain and nervous cell tissue. It accounts for up to 10% of all phospholipids in brain tissue. Its major functions is to regulate cell membrane integrity and fluidity. Trace amounts of phosphatidylserine are found in soy lecithin. Low levels of phosphatidylserine are associated with poor memory, depression and impaired cognitive function. Supplementation of phosphatidylserine have been shown in some studies and animals and humans to improve mood, memory and cognitive function. The recommended dose of phosphatidylserine is 100 milligrams 3 x per day. (17)

Essential fatty acid deficiency is a common nutritional deficiency in the elderly. Manifestations of EFA deficiency includes neurological signs such as poor memory and cognitive decline. Supplementation with a blend of EFA's seems to improve memory in some patients with Alzheimer's disease. This conjecture is interesting and further supports the theory that Alzheimer's disease is not just caused by acetylcholine deficiency. EFA's play such an important role in many facets of human biochemistry and EFA supplementation is simple and a cost effective measure for prevention and nutritional support. (18)

HORMONES

DHEA (Dehydroepiandosterone) is touted as a master steroid hormone of the human body. It is produces primarily in the adrenal glands. It is used to make a variety of sex hormones including estrogen, progesterone and testosterone and other steroid hormones including cortisone. Normal production of DHEA peaks at about age 25 to 30 years. It declines with age. Significant decline is experiences by some elderly individuals. (19) Supplementation may be beneficial in some individuals with poor memory and dementia. (20)

DMAE (Dimethylaminoethanol) is a natural precursor to acetylcholine. It is found in small amounts in seafood. It works slowly and has been shown to increase choline levels in the brain. Supplementation has been shown to improve some parameters of short and long term memory. It is also has been shown to improve moods and behavior. It is recommended for the treatment of hyperactivity in children. Large doses over time can produce agitation. The usually recommended dose of DMAE is 500 milligrams per day for children and 1000 milligrams per day for adults. (21)

BOTANICAL MEDICINES

One of the most popular, well studied and most effective geriatric medicines in the world is standardized Gingko biloba extract. In Europe Ginkgo biloba extract is one of the most frequently prescribed medicines. According to Julian Whitaker MD, some 10 million prescriptions for this medicine were written in 1989 by about 100,000 physicians. In France, 1.5% of all prescription sales are for ginkgo leaf extract. In Germany, 1.0% of all prescription sales are for ginkgo extract. (22)

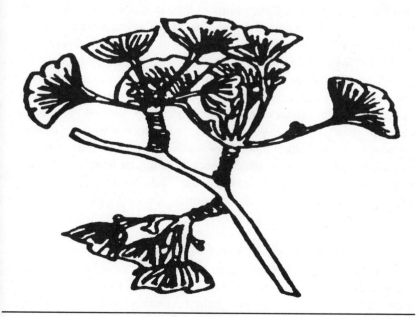

Gingko (Ginkgo biloba)

The pharmacologic activity of Ginkgo leaf is related to it's high content of terpenes, flavonoids, proanthocyanidins and flavoglycosides. Ginkgo biloba extract contains up to 24% flavoglycosides and is a widely available medicinal product throughout Europe. (23)

The pharmacologic effects of Ginkgo biloba can be summarized as follows: Ginkgo dilates blood vessels and as a result, increases blood flow and oxygen supply in the brain. Ginkgo decreases blood pressure. Ginkgo decreases atherosclerotic plaque formation in blood vessels. Ginkgo stabilizes the blood-brain barrier. Ginkgo acts as a free radical scavenger and prevents damage to cell membranes. Ginkgo increases the neurotransmitter, dopamine, which is believed to enhance nerve function in the brain. Ginkgo enhances the release of adrenaline from the adrenal glands and inhibits the enzyme responsible for it's breakdown. Ginkgo maintains venous tone. (24,25)

The clinical research with Ginkgo biloba extract is very encouraging. In one long term study, 112 geriatric patients with chronic cerebral insufficiency were treated with Ginkgo biloba extract (GBE) at 120 mg/day for one year. Results showed that the patients treated with GBE had significantly improved symptoms of brain blood flow insufficiency. Improved symptoms of headache, vertigo, tinnitus, short term memory, vigilance and mood disturbance were recorded. (25) In another study of 166 geriatric patients with vascular disorders due to aging, GBE improved their symptoms. The effects of GBE became significant after three months of administration. Functional changes in the EEG (Electroencephalogram) were noted and patients experienced improved mental alertness. (26) In another study with 20 patients with cerebral vascular insufficiency due to arteriosclerosis, dramatic improvement of cerebral blood flow was observed after only two weeks of GBE supplementation. Researchers in a study of Alzheimer's disease concluded that GBE appears to fulfill the conditions laid down by WHO (World Health Organization) concerning the development of a drug effective against cerebral aging. (27)

Ginkgo biloba is safe and non-toxic and few adverse side effects have been reported. Stomach upset and headache have been reported in some individuals who consumed GBE in doses of up to 600 mg/day. Consumption of the fruit and pulp of Ginkgo may cause allergic reactions including a topical red, inflamed, itchy rash. (28)

The doses of Ginkgo biloba extract most frequently used in clinical research is 120 mg/day. Doses of up to 600 mg/day have been consumed without adverse side effects. I usually recommend a dosage of 40 mg three times per day of Ginkgo biloba extract standardized for 24% Ginkgo heterosides.

Few other botanical medicines have the some clout and scientific documentation for treatment of poor memory and cognitive decline than Ginkgo biloba. One herbal extract that shows some promise is Panax ginseng. Panax ginseng is one of the most popular and most scientifically studied herbal medicine in the world. Well known as an adaptogen; to help improve our body's adaptation to stress, it also improves some parameters of memory and cognitive function. Supplementation of a standardized extract reflecting specific ginsensoside content, specifically RG1 fraction, has been shown to be beneficial for some patients with Alzheimer's disease. (29)

RECOMMENDATIONS: Daily unless otherwise stated

Folic acid..5-10 mg
Thiamine...5-10 mg
Vitamin B6...10-20 mg
Vitamin B12...50-100 mcg
Vitamin C...500-1000 mg
Vitamin E...200-400 IU
Zinc..25-50 mg
Lecithin (Phosphatidyl choline)................................5-25 gm
Phosphatidyl serine..300 mg
DMAE...750-1500 mg
Ginkgo biloba extract (24% heterosides)......................120 mg

REFERENCES

(1) Shaw DM et al: Senile Dementia and nutrition. Letter to the Editor. Brit. Med. J. 288:792-3, 1984
(2) Strachan RW and Henderson JG: Dementia and folate deficiency. Quart. J. Med. 36:189-204, 1967
(3) Bober MJ: Senile dementia and nutrition. Letter to the Editor. Brit. Med. J. 288:1234, 1984
(4) Mimori Y et al: Thiamine therapy in Alzheimer's disease. Metab. Brain Disp., Mar

11(1):89-94, 1996
(5) Keatings AMB et al: Vitamin B1, B2, B6 and C status in the elderly. Irish Med. J. 76:488-90, 1983
(6) Abalan F and Delile JM: B12 deficiency in presenile dementia. Letter to the Editor. Biol. Psychiat20(11):1251, 1985
(7) Schorah CJ et al: Human Nutr.: Clin Nutr. 37C:447-52, 1983
(8) Burns A and Holland T: Vitamin E deficiency. Letter to the Editor. Lancet. pp. 805-6, April 5, 1986
(9) Sylvester PE: Ageing in the mentally retarded. Scientific Studies in Mental Retardation. London, Macmillian, for the Royal Society of Medicine, pp. 259-77, 1984
(10) King RG: Do raised brain aluminum levels in Alzheimer's dementia contribute to cholinergic neuronal deficits? Med. Hypoth. 14:301-6, 1984
(11) Wilson SA: Progressive lenticular degeneration: A familial nervous disease associated with cirrhosis of the liver. Brain 34:296, 1912
(12) Schubert D and Chevion M: The role of iron in beta amyloid toxicity. Biochem. Biophys. Res. Commun., Nov. 13:216(2):702-7, 1996
(13) Mena I: Disorders of Mineral Metabolism. I. Trace Minerals, Academic Press, New York, NY. pp. 233-70, 1981
(14) Hullin RP: Serum zinc in psychiatric patients. Prog. Clin. Biol. Res. 129:197-206, 1983
(15) Rosenberg GS and Davis KL: The use of cholinergic precursors in neuropsychiatric diseases. Am. J. Clin. Nutr. 36:709-20, 1982
(16) Dysken M: A review of recent clinical trials in the treatment of Alzheimer's dementia. Psychiatric Annals 17(3)178, 1987
(17) Murray Michael T; Encyclopedia of Nutritional Supplements. Prima Publishing, Rocklin, CA., 1996
(18) Corrigan FM et al: Essential fatty acids in Alzheimer's disease. Ann. N.Y. Acad. Sci., 640:250-2, 1991
(19) Kalimi M and Regelson W: The Biological Role of Dehydroepiandosterone. de Gruyter, New York, NY, 1990
(20) Flood JF and Roberts E: Dehydroepiandosterone sulfate improves memory in aging mice. Brain Research 448:178-81, 1988.
(21) Amazing Medicines The Drug Companies Want You to Discover. University Medical Research Publishers, Tempe, Arizona 1993
(22) Foster S: Ginkgo. Botanical Series - 304. American Botanical Council, Austin, Texas, 1990.
(23) Briancon-Scheid F et al: HPLC separation and quantitative determination of biflavone in leaves from Ginkgo biloba. Planta Medica 49:204-7, 1983
(24) Pizzorno JE and Murray MT: A Textbook of Natural Medicine. JBC Publications, Seattle, Washington, 1985
(25) Voberg G: Ginkgo biloba extract (GBE): A long term study of chronic cerebral vascular insufficiency in geriatric patients. Clinical Trials J. 22:149-57, 1985
(26) Taillandier J et al: Treatment of cerebral ageing disorders with Ginkgo biloba extract. Presse Med. 15(31):1583-7, 1986
(27) Galley P et al: Tanakan et cerveau senile. Etude radiocirculographique. Bordeaux

Med. 10:171, 1977

(28) Becker LE et al: Ginkgo-tree dermatitis, stomatitis and proctitis. JAMA 231:1162-3, 1975

(29) Petkov VD et al: Memory effects of standardized Panax ginseng (G115), Ginkgo biloba (GK501) and their combination Gincosan (PHL-00701). Planta Medica, April: 59(2):106-114, 1993

CHAPTER 8

FIGHTING INFECTIONS NATURALLY

Except for dental caries the common cold is the most frequent infection experienced by human beings of all ages. The "average person" in North America is afflicted by 2 to 5 colds per year. This estimate translates to 100 million colds per year, approximately 250 million days of restricted activity, approximately 30 million lost days of work and an equal number of lost days of schooling. Cost estimates excluding expenses for worker absenteeism and professional health care, suggest that more than 3 billion dollars is spent on proprietary cold remedies and cold related analgesics per year. Clinical manifestations of the common cold include sore throat, nasal stuffiness, sneezing, watery discharge, malaise, slight fever and cough. Influenza or the flu, is an acute febrile disease that spreads rapidly as community outbreaks, disables large numbers of people and is usually not fatal. The uncomplicated form of influenza is a symptomatic illness with few localizing symptoms other than a severe headache. Clinical manifestations like the common cold include sore throat, fever, malaise, cough and muscle aches and pains. Grandmother's wisdom concerning treatment of the common cold with vitamin C, bedrest and chicken noodle soup is still the best approach that conventional medicine can offer. Both colds and influenza are caused by viruses and cannot be treated with antibiotics. Bacterial infections involving Streptococcus and Staphylococcus species are common in the upper respiratory tract and the skin. Bacterial infections are commonly treated with antibiotics. Safe and natural alternatives exist for the treatment of common infections.

DIET

Protein calorie malnutrition is associated with impaired immune function and increased susceptibility to infection. (1) A low fat, low cholesterol diet decreases susceptibility to infection. (2) Sugar impairs immune function. The ability of white blood cells to engulf bacteria is significantly depressed with sugar consumption. (3)

NUTRIENTS

Folic acid deficiency is associated with impaired host resistance and depressed immune function. (2)

Pantothenic acid (Vitamin B5) deficiency depresses antibody response to various infectious agents, but has not been shown to impair cell-mediated immunity. (2)

Pyridoxine (Vitamin B6) deficiency inhibits cell-mediated immune functions, as well as antibody response. (4)

Riboflavin (Vitamin B2) if deficient impairs immunity. (2)

Vitamin A deficiency impairs immune function and is associated with decreased cellular immune response to foreign infection. (5) Vitamin A excess alters white blood cell response to infectious agents and antibody response and may diminish host susceptibility to infection. (2)

Vitamin B12 deficiency can lead to pernicious anemia and impairs white blood cell function. (6)

Bacterial infection can reduce cellular uptake of Vitamin C. (7) White blood cell concentrations of vitamin C are significantly decreased in the common cold. Vitamin C deficiency impairs the function of white blood cells to surround and eliminate foreign agents. Supplementation may reduce the severity and duration and possibly the incidence of the common cold and certain bacterial infections. (8)

Vitamin E deficiency is associated with increased infections due to decreased membrane related chemotaxis and decreased white blood cell function (9)

Copper deficiency may be associated with increased susceptibility to infection due to impairment of immune function and copper excess may increase susceptibility to infection. (1,2)

Iron deficiency may be associated with increased susceptibility to infection while excess supplementation can increase bacterial growth and replications and release of certain exotoxins. (2)

Magnesium and phosphorus deficiency may hinder immune response. (2,10)

Selenium is associated with the oxidative functions believed to be important for killing bacteria and deficiency may impair immune function. (10)

Zinc deficiency may be associated with impaired immune responses. (1) Zinc supplementation improves T-cell function. (11) Supplementation may be effective in reducing the onset, severity and duration of the common cold. (12) Excess zinc however, impairs immune responses. (13)

Essential fatty acids, including the oils of evening primrose, fish and linseed are rich in linoleic, linolenic and eicosapentaenoic acid, have antibacterial, antifungal and antiviral effects. (14)

OTHER FACTORS

Lead and cadmium toxicities have adverse effects of host resistance to bacterial and viral infections. (15)

Decreased stomach acidity increases both susceptibility and severity of bacterial and parasitic infections. (16)

Acidophyllin, the antibacterial component of Lactobacillus acidophillus, causes inhibition of common bacterial pathogens. (17)

BOTANICAL MEDICINES

Garlic (Allium sativa) is a common, strong scented perennial herb native to Europe, central Asia and has been naturalized in North America and is cultivated worldwide. The fresh or dehydrated bulb has been used medicinally for thousands of years. Garlic bulb contains 0.1 to 0.36% volatile oil consisting of allicin and other sulphur containing compounds. (18) Garlic has been traditionally used to treat coughs, colds, influenza, bronchitis, toothache and many other ailments. In the People's Republic of China cloves of garlic are eaten and concentrated extracts are given intravenously to treat cryptococcal meningitis. Garlic has been used to treat various bacterial, fungal and viral infections. Grandmother's wisdom using garlic to treat colds, influenza and other infections is supported by scientific research.

Garlic is a broad spectrum antibiotic that rivals penicillin. Antibiotic effects of garlic have been demonstrated against Staphylococcus species, Streptococcus species, Brucella, Klebsiella, Proteus, E.coli, Vibrio cholerae, Salmonella, Bacillus, and Pseudomonas. Antifungal activity of garlic has been demonstrated against Candida species, Trichophyton, Microsporum, Cryptococcus and Epidermophyton and Histoplasm. (19) Antiviral activity of garlic has been demonstrated by the Shanghai Tenth Pharmaceutical Factory against Influenza B and herpes simplex viruses. (20) Based on various studies, the antimicrobial activity of garlic is due to the sulphur-containing volatile oils. (19) Garlic is a potent broad spectrum antibiotic against bacteria, fungi and viruses. Garlic is virtually non-toxic and safe to use, although some allergic reactions including contact dermatitis and stomach upset have been reported.

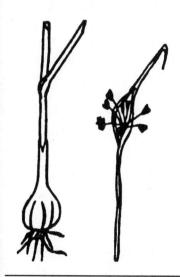 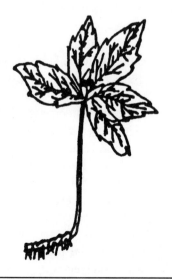

Garlic (Allium sativum)   Goldenseal (Hydrastis canadensis)

Goldenseal (Hydrastis canadensis) is a small perennial plant growing up to 30 centimeters in height in damp woods and meadows of eastern United States and Canada. Goldenseal is cultivated in parts of the west coast. Goldenseal has a rough, wrinkled root with a distinctive odor and bitter taste. The Cherokee Indians used goldenseal root to treat skin ulcers and arrow wounds. The root has also been used traditionally as an antiseptic, diuretic, hemostatic, laxative and tonic and to relieve inflamed mucous membranes. (21)

Isoquinoline alkaloids have been isolated from goldenseal root and are responsible for a majority of this plant's medicinal actions. Alkaloids isolated include hydrastine (1.5 to 4.0%), berberine (0.5 to 6.0%), berberastine (2.0 to 3.0%) and other related alkaloids are present at lower concentrations. (22)

Berberine and the other alkaloids of Hydrastis have demonstrated antimicrobial effects against bacteria, fungi and protozoa. Antibacterial activity has been demonstrated against Staphylococcus species, Streptococcus species, Corynebacterium diptheriae, Vibrio cholerae, Shigella, Klebsiella pneumoniae, Bacillus subtilus, E. coli, Pseudomonas, Salmonella and Proteus species. Antifungal activity has been demonstrated against Candida, Cryptococcus, Microsporum, Sporothrix, and Trichophytons. Antiprotozoal activity has been demonstrated against Entamoeba histolytica, Leishmania donovani, Mycobacterium tuberculosis, Xanthomonas citri and Giardia lamblia. (23) Bereberine has demonstrated effective treatment of gastrointestinal disorders caused by E. coli, Shigella dysynteriae, Salmonella, Klebsiella, Giardia lamblia, Vibrio cholerae and Entamoeba histolytica. (23) Berberine is particularly effective in treating acute diarrhea caused by these organisms and the optimal pH for its action is pH 8. (24) The antimicrobial mechanism of berberine has not been completely elucidated. Berberine inhibits DNA replication and protein synthesis. Berberine also acts directly on ribosomes and renders ribosomal RNA susceptible to hydrolysis by ribonuclease enzymes which are found in association with isolated bacterial ribosomes. Berberine alters fatty acid composition in bacteria and inhibits the formation of cholera toxins and berberine may exert toxic effects by acting as a membrane poison. (23) Berberine has been shown to stimulate phagocytic activity of macrophages and increases blood supply to the spleen. (25) Berberine has also displayed antipyretic activity. (26)

Berberine and other alkaloids isolated from Hydrastis show broad range antimicrobial activity against various bacteria, fungi and protozoa. 356 patients with severe diarrhea, of which 92 were positive and 264 were negative for Vibrio cholerae, were treated with a 15 mg dose of berberine three to four times a day. After 3 days of treatment significant improvement was observed as measured by decreased mortality rate, duration of diarrhea and fluid intake. (27)

Berberine and the other alkaloids of Hydrastis canadensis are safe and non-toxic. Berberine and berberine containing plants are not recommended during pregnancy. (25)

RECOMMENDATIONS: Daily unless otherwise stated

Folic acid	400-800 mcg
Pantothenic Acid	500 mg
Pyridoxine	25-50 mg
Riboflavin	10-25 mg
Vitamin A	10,000-20,000 IU
Vitamin C	2000-5000 mg
Vitamin E	200-400 IU
Copper	2-4 mg
Iron	10-25 mg
Magnesium	400-800 mg
Phosphorus	800 mg
Selenium	200-400 mcg
Zinc	25-50 mg
Essential oils	3-6 gm
HCl supplements	3-6 caps
Allium sativa (Fresh Garlic)	10-30 gm
Hydrastis canadensis (4:1)	500-1000 mg

REFERENCES

(1) Chandra RK: Trace element regulation of immunity and infection. J. Am. Coll. Nutr. 4(1):5-16, 1985
(2) Beisel WR: Single nutrients and immunity. Am. J. Clin. Nutr. 35:417-68 (suppl.), 1982
(3) Sanchez A et al: Role of sugars in human neutrophilic phagocytosis. Am. J. Clin. Nutr. 26:180, 1973
(4) Axelrod AE et al: Relationship of pyridoxine to immunological phenomena. Vitam.

Horm. 22:591-607, 1964
(5) Hof H: Vitamin A, the "anti-infective" vitamin? MMW 118(46):1485-88, 1976
(6) Kaplan SS et al: Effect of vitamin B12 and folic acid deficiencies on neutrophil function. Blood 47:801-5, 1976
(7) Wilson CWM: Clinical pharmacological aspects of ascorbic acid. Ann. N.Y. Acad. Sci. 258:355-76, 1975
(8) Baird IM et al: The effects of ascorbic acid and flavonoids on the occurence of symptoms normally associated with the common cold. Am. J. Clin. Nutr. 32:1686-90, 1979
(9) Baehner RL et al: Role of membrane vitamin E and cytoplasmic glutathione in the regulation of phagocytic functions of neutrophils and monocytes. Am. J. Pediatr. Hematol. Oncol. 1(1):71-76, 1979
(10) Miller ER: Mineral X disease interactions. J. Anim. Sci. 60(6):1500-7, 1985
(11) Duchateau J et al: Influence of oral zinc supplementation on the lymphocyte response to mitogens of normal subjects. Am. J. Clin. Nutr. 34:88-93, 1981
(12) Eby GA et al: Antimicrobial Agents & Chemotherapy 25:20-24, January, 1984
(13) Chandra RK: Excessive intake of zinc impairs immune responses. JAMA 252(11):1443-46, 1984
(14) Das UN: Antibiotic-like action of essential fatty acids. Can. Med. Assoc. J. 132:1350, 1985
(15) Gainer JH: Effects of heavy metals and of deficiency of zinc on mortality rates in mice infected with encephalomyocarditis virus, Am. J. Vet. Res. 38:869-72, 1977
(16) Giannella RA et al: Influence of gastric acidity on bacterial and parasitic enteric infections. ANN. Int. Med. 78:271-76, 1973
(17) Shanhani KM et al: Role of dietary lactobacilli in gastrointestinal microecology. AM. J. Clin. Nutr. 33:2448-2457, 1980
(18) Block E: The Chemistry of Garlic and Onions. Scientific American, pp. 114-119, March 1985
(19) Adetumbi MA et al: Allium sativum (Garlic) - A natural antibiotic, Medical Hypotheses 12:227-37, 1985
(20) Tsai Y et al: Antiviral properties of Garlic: In vitro effects of Influenza B, Herpes simplex and Coxsackie viruses, Planta Medica No. 5, 1985
(21) Duke JA: Handbook of Medicinal Herbs. CRC Press. Boca Raton, FL., 287-8, 1985
(22) Leung AY: Encyclopedia of Common Natural Ingredients Used in Food, Drugs, and Cosmetics. John Wiley & Sons, New York, NY. pp. 189-90, 1980
(23) Hahn FE et al: Berberine. Antibiotics 3:577-88, 1976(24) Amin AH et al: Berberine sulfate: Antimicrobial activity, bioassay and mode of action. Can. J. Microbiol. 15:1067-76, 1969
(25) Sabir M et al: Study of some pharmacologic actions of berberin. Ind. J. Physiol. Pharm. 15:111-32, 1971
(26) Sabir M et al: Further studies on pharmacology of berberine. Ind. J. Physiol. Pharmacol. 22-23, 1978
(27) Sack RB et al: Berberine inhibits intestinal secretory response of vibrio cholerae toxins and Escherichia coli enterotoxins. Infect. Immun. 35:471-5, 1982

CHAPTER 9

HAVING A HEALTHY LIVER

The liver is one of the largest and the most metabolically active organs in the human body. The liver is an extremely complex organ and it has been estimated that over 500 different metabolic functions occur within each liver cell. These functions involve such broad categories as intermediate metabolism of carbohydrates, proteins and fats; synthesis of proteins and a host of enzymes; production of bile; detoxification and removal of foreign material and toxins, such as bacteria, drugs, alcohol and other noxious substances; storage of protein, glycogen, vitamins and minerals; and many other functions too numerous to list here. The liver is one of the most frequently damaged organs in the body and it is indeed fortunate that it has an incredible regeneration capacity. It has also been experimentally shown that only 10% of the liver is required to maintain normal liver function. The diseases that affect the liver include both acute and chronic hepatits, fatty liver degeneration, cirrhosis and liver cancer. Natural therapies are available that help the liver function and prevent liver damage.

DIET

A diet high in sugar and refined carbohydrates is associated with elevated liver enzymes (SGOT and SGPT) which are associated with liver damage. A diet low in sugar and refined carbohydrates is associated with decreased liver enzymes and decreased serum triglycerides. (1)

NUTRIENTS

Vitamin B12 supplementation is beneficial in viral hepatitis. (2) Supplementation with vitamin B12 brought about a rapid return of appetite and liver size to normal in patients with viral hepatitis. (3) Supplementation with Vitamin B12 and Folic Acid was associated with a subjective improvement in the state of the patients and a shorter duration of illness. (3)

Vitamin C supplementation may expediate patient recovery time. Patients treated with 400 to 600 mg/kg of Vitamin C were back to work 3 to 7 days following treatment. (4) 245 children with viral hepatitis who received 10 grams of Vitamin C daily experienced rapid recovery of their illness. (5)

In one study, 338 patients with chronic hepatitis received either 1.5 gram of catechin daily for two weeks followed by 2.25 gram for 14 weeks or placebo. Catechin consists of bioflavonoids derived from the plants Uncaria gambir or Acacia catechu. Patients treated with catechin displayed lower liver enzyme and liver function tests than those patients treated with placebo. (6)

BOTANICAL MEDICINES

Artichoke (Cynara scolymus) is a large thistle-like perennial herb that grows up to 1 meter tall and is native to southern Europe, North Africa and the Canary Islands. The immature flowerheads with fleshy tracts are eaten as a vegetable. Ingredients in artichoke include up to 2.0% diphenolic derivatives including cynarin and scolumoside. (7) Artichoke has been reported to have stimulant, choleretic and diuretic properties. Cynarin and scolymoside increase bile secretion from the liver. (7) Cynarin has also been reported to reduce blood cholesterol and triglycerides. Cynara extracts exert a positive influence on liver cell regeneration. (8) In one controlled study with cynarin in the treatment of hypercholesterolemia, there was a significant reduction of cholesterol levels. The researchers concluded that cynara is effective in the prophylaxis and treatment of arteriosclerotic disease. (9)

Dandelion (Taraxacum officinale) literally means "lion's tooth" and is a common garden weed. Dandelion is mentioned as early as the 10th century by Arab physicians who used the plant for medicinal purposes. The bitter greens are used in raw salads, in wine making or cooked like spinach. The taproot is roasted and used to brew a coffee-like beverage said to lack the stimulant properties of coffee. Dandelion contains small amounts of alkaloids, glycosides, tannins and mineral salts. (7) Other components include taraxerol, choline and inulin. The plant contains the bitter principle taraxacin and appears to be a good source of Vitamin A. (7) Studies involving both animal and human subjects have demonstrated that dandelion increases the flow of bile from the liver and gall bladder. Dandelion exhibits a choleretic effect, increasing both production and secretion of bile from the liver and a cholagogue effect, increasing contraction of the gall bladder which releases stored bile into the intestinal tract. (21) Dandelion extracts enhance bile discharge and are indicated in inflammatory liver conditions.

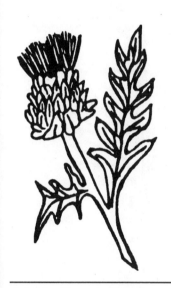 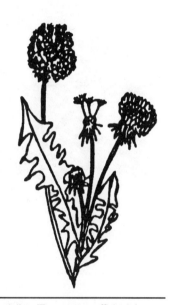

Artichoke (Cynara scolymus)   Dandelion (Taraxacum officinale)

Milk thistle (Silybum marianum) grows from 1 to 3 meters in height and has large prickly leaves and attractive red and purple flowers. Milk thistle is indigenous to Kashmir and is also found in Europe and North America from Canada to Mexico. The ancient Greeks used the plant medicinally and named it "silybum" meaning thistle. During the middle ages monks introduced the plant into Europe and regarded the plant with mythical and religious adoration. Milk thistle has been use in folk medicine to treat liver disorders including jaundice, gallstones, peritonitis, hemorrhage, bronchitis and varicose veins. In the 18th century milk thistle was the treatment of choice in liver disorders. The seeds, leaves and fruit have been used for medicinal purposes. (10)

The crude extract obtained from milk thistle was originally termed silymarin. Silymarin represents a mixture of flavonoid compounds called flavonolignans. Three major flavonolignans identified in silymarin include silybin, silydianin and silychristin. While these flavonoids are found in leaves and fruit, they are found in highest concentration in the ripe seeds. The ripe seeds contain 4.0 to 6.0% silymarin. Silymarin has been identified as the active ingredient in milk thistle responsible for its medicinal effects. Silybum marianum extracts are usually standardized to contain 70 to 80% silymarin content. (10)

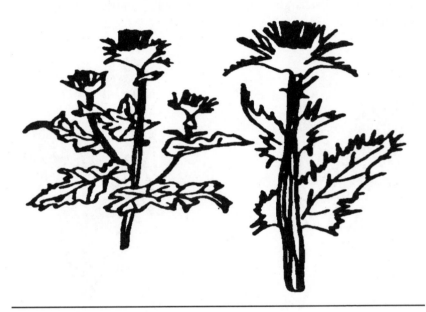

Milk thistle (Silybum marianum)

The pharmacologic action of silymarin is specific to the liver. Silymarin exhibits potent anti-hepatotoxic effects when the liver is insulted by toxins including carbon tetrachloride, thioacetamide, galactosamine and heavy metals. (11,12,13). Silymarin protects the liver from the potentially fatal damage caused by ingestion of poisonous mushrooms. Aminita phalloides is commonly known as the deathcap mushroom and is responsible for up to 50% of fatalities due to mushroom poisoning. Aminita mushroom produces signs of toxicity 8 to 10 hours following consumption and can result in death 30 to 40 hours later. Aminita toxin produces damage to liver cells by increasing the permeability of liver membranes which results in cell destruction and by inhibiting the polymerase B enzyme in the cell nucleus which inhibits protein synthesis. Silymarin is capable of antagonizing the effects of aminita toxin at these two levels. Silymarin administered to mice up to 30 minutes after aminita poisoning showed no signs of liver damage. (11) It has been postulated that silymarin exerts its effects by stabilizing liver cell membranes preventing toxins from entering the cell. Silymarin also stimulates protein synthesis and thereby promotes regeneration of liver cells. (14) Silymarin inhibits the enzyme lipoxygenase which inhibits the production of inflammatory products including leukotrienes. (15) Silymarin also is a potent antioxidant, exerting greater antioxidant activity than Vitamin E. (16) The pharmacologic actions of silymarin can be summarized as follows:

Stabilizes and strengthens liver cell membranes and thereby prevents toxins from penetrating liver cells.2. Increases the rate of protein synthesis and thereby increases regeneration of liver cells.3, Acts as an antioxidant and free radical scavenger.4. Inhibits the production of the enzyme lipoxygenase involved in the productions of the damaging leukotrienes.

One hundred and twenty-nine patients with a number of different liver disorders including, toxic damage, cirrhosis, fatty degeneration and chronic hepatitis were treated with milk thistle extract. Significant improvements in the condition of treated subjects were observed. (17) Liver enzymes (SGPT, SGOT) were monitored and returned to normal faster in treated subjects. Liver size decreased and subjective improvement in symptoms and digestive function was noted. In a clinical trial of 205 individuals with aminita toxicity, 46 patients died, but all individuals treated with silymarin survived. (18) Researchers concluded that administration of silymarin 48 hours following ingestion, at a dose of 20 to 50 mg/kg/day,was an effective prophylactic measure against severe liver damage. Another study involving 55 patients with severe aminita poisoning who were treated with 20 mg/kg of silymarin showed good results and none of the treated patients died. (19) Thirty-six patients with liver cirrhosis, both acute and chronic hepatitis, were treated with milk thistle extract. Inflammation and cirrhosis diminished or disappeared with administration of milk thistle extract over several months. (20)

No adverse effects of both acute and long term administration of silymarin use have been reported. The long term safety and the use of these extracts during pregnancy remains to be established. (11)

RECOMMENDATIONS: Daily unless otherwise stated

Vitamin B12...100 mcg
Folic Acid..40-60 mg
Vitamin C...3000-5000 mg
Catechin...1000-2000 mg
Cynara scolymus (4:1)...500-1000 mg
Silybum Marianum (10:1)..400-800 mg
Taraxacum officinalis (4:1)..250-500 mg

REFERENCES

(1) Porikos KP et al: Diet-induced changes in serum transaminase and triglyceride levels in healthy adult men. Role of sucrose and excess calories. Am. J. Med. 75:624, 1983

(2) Jain ASC et al: Observations on the therapeutic value of intravenous B12 in infective hepatitis. J. Indian Med. Assoc. 35:502-5, 1960

(3) Campbell RE et al: Vitamin B12 in the treatment of viral hepatitis. Am. J. Med. Sci. 224:252, 1952

(4) Klenner FR: Observations on the dose of administration of ascorbic acid when employed beyond the range of a vitamin in human pathology. J. Applied Nutr. 23(3&4):61-88, 1961

(5) Baetgen D: Results of the treatment of epidemic hepatitis in children with high doses of ascorbic acid in the years 1957-1958. Medisinische Monatschrift 15:30-36, 1961

(6) Suzuki H et al: Cianidanol therapy for Hbe-antigen positive chronic hepatitis: A multicentre, double-blind study. Liver 6:35, 1986

(7) Leung AY: Encyclopedia of Common Natural Ingredients Used in Food, Drug, and Cosmetics. John Wiley & Sons, New York, NY. 1980

(8) Pristautz H: Cynarin in the modern treatment of hyperlipidemias. Weiner Medizinische Wocheschrift 1223:705-9, 1975

(9) Maros T et al: The effects of Cynara scolymus extracts on the regeneration of the rat liver. Arzneim-Forsch. 16:127-9, 1966

(10) Wagner H: Antihepatotoxic flavonoids. In: Plant Flavonoids in Biology and Medicine: Biochemical, Pharmacological, and Structure-Activity relationshps. Edited by Cody V et al. Alan R liss, Inc, New York, NY, pp. 545-58, 1986

(11) Hahn G et al: The pharmacology and toxicology of Silymarin; the antihepatotoxic principles of Silybum marianum. Arzneim-Forsch. 18(6):698-704, 1968

(12) Desplaces A et al: The Effects of Silymarin on Experimental Phalloidine Poisoning. Arzneim-Forsch. 25(1):89-96, 1975

(13) Strubelt O et al: The influence of silybin on the hepatotoxic and hypoglycemic effects of praseodymium and other lanthanides. Arzneim-Forsch. 30:1690-94, 1980

(14) Sonnenbichler J et al: Stimulatory effect of silibinin on the DNA synthesis in partially hepatectomized rat livers: non-response in hepatoma and other malignant cell lines. Bichem. Pharm. 35:538-41, 1986

(15) Fiebrich F et al: Silymarin, an inhibitor of of lipoxygenase. Experentia 35:148-150, 1979

(16) Adzet T: Polyphenolic compounds with biological and pharmacological activity. Herbs Spices Medicinal Plants 1:167-84, 1986

(17) Schopen RD et al: Searching for a new therapeutic principle. Experience with hepatic therapeutic legalon. Med Welt 20:888-93, 1969

(18) Florsheim GL et al: Die klinische knollenblaitterpilzvergiftung (aminita phalloides): prognotische faktoren und therapeitosche massnahmen. Schwiez. Medizinische Wochenschrift 112:1164-77, 1982

(19) Boari C et al: Occupational toxic liver diseases. Therapeutic effects of Silymarin. Min. Med. 72:2679-88, 1981

(20) Schilder M: Silymarin in der klinischen pruefung. Ein bericht ueber 36 faelle von verschiedenen leberkrankheiten in laegsschnittuntersuchungen. Therapiewoche 20:3444, 1970

(21) The Lawrence Review of Natural Products: Dandelion. Pharmaceutical Information Associates, Ltd., Levittown, Pennsylvania, December, 1987

CHAPTER 10

HEALING STOMACH ULCERS

Peptic ulcers, involving the stomach and duodenum, occur in 5 to 10% of the North American population and involve twice as many males as females. The illness is considered a disease of young and middle-aged adults. The cause of ulcer formation is rarely due to excessive secretion of stomach acid, primarily hydrochloric acid, as is assumed by many. Most cases represent an imbalance between acid, enzymes and other potentially damaging agents and factors that act to protect mucousal integrity. The protective lining of the stomach, called a mucous membrane, consists of a group of sugars known as polysaccharides and proteins and enzymes, that line the inner stomach wall and normally prevents stomach acid from digesting through the stomach wall. Ulcers are caused when there is a weakening of the mucous membrane and stomach acid is allowed to digest through the membrane and irritates the stomach wall.

Conventional therapy is aimed at reducing stomach acid secretions. Tagamet (Cimetidine) and Zantac (Ranitidine) are two of the most common drugs routinely prescribed in ulcer therapy. They are histamine-2 receptor antagonists and they markedly inhibit hydrochloric acid secretion. Histamine is usually released from nerve endings that supply parietal cells of the stomach, which stimulates these cells to produce hydrochloric acid. Histamine-2 receptor antagonists bind to the cellular receptor on the parietal cells without producing any physiological effect. The net result is that production of hydrochloric acid in the stomach is markedly decreased. However, decreasing excessive stomach acid is not usually the problem. Common side effects caused by both drugs include drowsiness, lethargy, dizziness, diarrhea, rash, and liver damage. Natural, safe and very effective alternatives to conventional therapy exist and should be considered in ulcer therapy treatment.

DIET

A diet high in fiber helps ulcers heal at a higher rate than a low fiber diet. (1) Patients on a high fiber diet improved symptomatically and suffered less relapse than those patients on a low fiber diet. (2) Snacking and foods found to be irritating to the stomach should be avoided. (3) Frequent milk ingestion should also be avoided. It is a popular misconception that milk decreases stomach acidity and should be consumed in larger quantities if a patient has an ulcer. This is however, a popular misconception. Milk has only a transient neutralizing effect on stomach acidity, followed by an increase in acid secretion. (4) Alcohol, coffee, tea and other caffeine-containing foods, stimulate stomach acid secretion and should be avoided. (5,6) Patients on a diet low in refined carbohydrates including sugar, had greater symptomatic improvement than those patients on a high refined carbohydrate diet. Sugar may be irritating to the stomach and sugar consumption should be decreased. (7)

NUTRIENTS

Bioflavonoids inhibit histamine release and supplementation with bioflavonoids reduced histamine levels in stomach tissue. Decreased histamine levels means decreased hydrochloric acid levels in the stomach. (8)

Pyridoxine (Vitamin B6) may be deficient in patients with peptic ulcers and supplementation may help to heal stress-induced ulcers. (9)

Vitamin A supplementation significantly reduced both the number and size of stress ulcers. (10)

Vitamin C levels is lower in patients with peptic ulcers and has been correlated with gastrointestinal hemorrhage. (11) Vitamin C supplementation may also improve the healing time of the ulcer. (12)

Vitamin E may provide protection against stress related ulcer. (13)

Zinc supplementation may inhibit the release of vasoactive

substances from stomach cells, thereby preventing changes in circulation known to cause mucousal irritation. (14)

Glutamine supplementation 400 mg four times a day, one hour before meals and before retiring for bed provides beneficial results. (15)

Food sensitivities have been implicated in the occurrence of peptic ulcers and elimination diets provide effective relief of ulcer symptoms. (16)

BOTANICAL MEDICINES

Fresh cabbage juice has been used for centuries to treat stomach and duodenal ulcers. The effectiveness of cabbage juice in the treatment of ulcers has been attributed to its high glutamine content. Patients who consumed one liter of fresh cabbage juice per day showed remarkable improvement in the healing time of the ulcers. Glutamine is believed to be involved in the synthesis of mucous which lines the stomach and protects the stomach from the harsh effects of acid. (17)

Plantain banana has also been used to decrease ulcer formation and enhance ulcer healing time. Unripe plantain banana increases mucousal resistance to factors that induce ulcer formation. (18)

Licorice (Glycyrrhiza glabra) a perennial plant that grows 1 to 2 meters in height, is native to Asia, Europe and parts of the Middle East. Licorice used primarily for its roots and rhizomes is widely used as a condiment to flavor candies and tobacco. Roots contain glycyrrhizin which is 50 times sweeter than sugar. It is interesting to note that most licorice candy doesn't contain any licorice at all, but rather anise oil. Licorice root was found in King Tut's tomb. Licorice is considered a demulcent, an expectorant, estrogenic and a laxative. The root and its derivatives have been used for centuries to treat a wide array of illness, including asthma, bronchitis, colds, diabetes, inflammation, emollient, constipation, eye pain, wounds and other illnesses. Licorice has also been used successfully to treat gastric and duodenal ulcers with remarkable effectiveness. (19)

The active ingredients in licorice root include triterpenoid glycosides known as glycyrrhizin, ranging at levels of 1.0 to 27%, averaging about 10 to 16%. Licorice root also contains flavonoids, isoflavonoids, sterols, volatile oil, tannins, saponins and sugars. Glycyrrhizin is 50 to 100 times sweeter than sugar. (20)

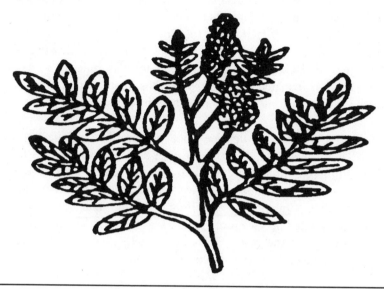

Licorice (Glycyrrhiza glabra)

Glycyrrhizin was originally thought to be the only active ingredient responsible for this plant's remarkable effectiveness in treating peptic ulcers. However, excessive intake of glycyrrhizin causes a condition known as pseudo-aldosteronism, marked by electrolyte imbalance, swelling, edema and hypertension. (21) In response to these adverse side effects, glycyrrhizin was removed from the plant extract giving rise to a substance known as Deglycyrrhizinated Licorice root or DGL. DGL has demonstrated remarkable effectiveness in treating peptic ulcers without the side effects caused by ingestion of glycyrrhizin. (22) DGL is as effective as Tagamet or Zantac and unlike these drugs DGL has a unique mechanism of action. DGL increases the number of mucous producing cells lining the stomach, increases the lifespan of these cells, increases the quality and quantity of mucous produced and decreases stomach mucousal blood flow, thought to play an important role against mucousal injury. (23)

In clinical studies, DGL accelerates the healing time of peptic ulcers and doesn't display the side effects encountered with use of raw licorice root preparations and conventional drugs. In one double-blind study, 16 patients received 760 mg of DGL three times a day versus 17 patients who received an equal amount of placebo for four weeks. Stomach ulcer size was significantly reduced in the 16 DGL treated patients and radiologically disappeared in 6 of the DGL treated patients. (24) In another study, 40 patients received 3.0 grams of DGL daily for 8 weeks or 4.5 grams of DGL daily for 16 weeks. All 40 patients showed significant improvement usually within 5 to 7 days following initial treatment with DGL. (25) DGL in tablet form is superior to capsule form. Degylyrrhizinated licorice tablets, has demonstrated remarkable effectiveness in treating both stomach and duodenal ulcers.

Glycyrrhizin in licorice root preparations mimics adrenal cortical hormones including the hormone aldosterone. Aldosterone causes fluid retention. Glycyrrhizin can also cause excessive fluid retention leading to a condition known as pseudo-aldosteronism, marked by electrolyte imbalance, swelling, edema and hypertension. Deglycyrrhizinated licorice root preparations have glycyrrhizin removed and doesn't cause the side effects noted with glycyrrhiziningestion. Deglycyrrhizinated licorice extracts are safe and no-toxic. (26)

RECOMMENDATIONS: Daily unless otherwise stated

Bioflavonoids..1-2 gm
Vitamin B6...25-50 mg
Vitamin A..50,000 IU
Vitamin C...1000-3000 mg
Vitamin E..400-800 IU
Zinc (Zinc Sulphate)..500 mg
Glutamine..1000-2000 mg
Cabbage Juice...1 litre
Plantain Banana..2-4
Glycyrrhiza glabra (DGL)..750-1500 mg

REFERENCES

(1) Rydning A et al: Prophylactic effect of dietary fiber in duodenal ulcer disease. Lancet 2:736-39, 1982
(2) Rydning A et al: Fiber diet and antacids in the short-term treatment of duodenal ulcer. Scand. J. Gastroenterol. 20(9):1078-82
(3) Welsh JD: Diet therapy of peptic ulcer disease. Gastroenterology 72:740-45, 1977
(4) Ippoliti AF et al: The effects of various forms of milk on gastric-acid secretion. Ann.

Intern. Med. 84:286-89, 1976

(5) Lenz HJ et al: Wine and five percent ethanol are potent stimulants of gastric acid secretion in human. Gastroenterology 85(5):1082-87, 1983

(6) Dubey P et al: Dig. Dis. & Sci. 29(3):202-06, 1984

(7) Yudkin J: Eating and ulcers. Letter to the editor. Brit. Med. J. February 16, 1980, pp. 483-84

(8) Amella M et al: Inhibition of mast cell histamine release by flavonoids and bioflavonoids. Planta Medica 51:16-20, 1985

(9) Sanderson CR et al: Serum pyridoxal in patients with active peptic ulcerations. Gut 16:177, 1975

(10) Patty I et al: Controlled trials of vitamin A in gastric ulcer. Lancet 2:876, 1982

(11) Russell RL et al: Ascorbic acid levels in leucocytes of patients with gastrointestinal hemorrhage. Lancet 2:603-6, 1968

(12) Debray C et al: Treatment of gastro-duodenal ulcers with large doses of ascorbic acid. Semaine Therapeutique (Paris) 44:393-8, 1968

(13) Kangas J et al: Am. J. Clin. Nutr., September 1972

(14) Frommer DJ: The healing of gastric ulcers with zinc sulphate. Med. J. Aust. 2:793, 1975

(15) Shive W et al: Glutamine in treatment of peptic ulcer. Texas State J. of Med. November, 1957, pp. 840-43

(16) Siegel J: Immunologic approach to the treatment and prevention of gastrointestinal ulcers. Ann. Allergy 38:27-41, 1977

(17) Cheney G: Rapid healing of peptic ulcer in patients receiving fresh cabbage juice. Cal. Med. 70:10-14, 1949

(18) Goel RK et al: The effect of biological variables on the anti-ulcerogenic effect of vegetable plantain banana. Planta Medica 2:85-88, 1985

(19) Leung AY: Encyclopedia of Common Natural Ingredients Used in Food, Durgs, and Cosmetics. John Wiley &Sons, New York, NY, 1980

(20) Tyler V et al: Pharmacognosy 8th ed., Lea & Febiger, Philadelphia, Pennsylvania, pp 69-70, 1981

(21) Epstein M et al: Effects of eating liquorice on the renin-angiotensin-aldosterone axis in normal subjects. Br. Med. J. 1:488-90, 1977

(22) Rees WDR et al: Effect of deglycyrrhizinated liquorice on gastric mucosal damage by aspirin. Scand. J. Gastroent. 14:605-7, 1962

(23) Morgan AG et al: Comparison between cimetidine and Caved-S in the treatment of gastric ulcerations and subsequent maintenance therapy. Gut 23:545-51, 1982

(24) Turpie AG et al: Clinical trials of deglycyrrhizinated liquorice in gastric ulcer. Gut 10:299-303, 1969

(25) Tewari SN et al: Deglycyrrhizinated licorice in duodenal ulcer disease. Practitioner 210:820-5, 1972

(26) Baron J et al: Metabolic studies, aldosterone secretion rate and plasma renin after carbonoxolone sodium as biogastrone. Br. Med. J. 2:793-5, 1969

CHAPTER 11

HEALTHY HEART TONIC

Heart disease is the leading cause of premature death before the age of 65 years. One of every three men and one of every ten women can expect to develop some form of heart disease before the age of 60 years. Major diseases of the heart and blood vessels were responsible for an estimated one million deaths, about half of all deaths in North America. In 1986, about 1.5 million persons experienced a heart attack in North America and of whom 500,000 died. A heart attack results from the formation of a blood clot or thrombus within a coronary artery and may shut off or occlude the blood flow to a section of the heart. The consequence of lack of blood flow to a section of the heart can result in permanent damage or injury to heart muscle. Risk factors for developing heart disease include elevated blood pressure, elevated cholesterol (especially LDL cholesterol) and triglycerides, family history of heart disease, glucose intolerance including diabetes mellitus, cigarette smoking, lack of physical activity, obesity and psychosocial factors including anxiety, life events and stress. In addition, Type A behavior characterized by extreme competiveness, impatience, time urgency, striving for achievement, abrupt, tense speech and movement, is a risk factor for developing heart disease. Natural therapies exist that can be used in conjunction with conventional therapies to help the heart function and aid in the prevention of heart disease.

DIET

In order to prevent cardiovascular disease, the Nutrition Committee of the American Heart Association has developed the following dietary guidelines for healthy adults. (1)

- Total fat intake should be less than 30% of calories.
- Saturated fat intake should be less than 10% of calories.

- Carbohydrate intake should constitute 50% or more of calories, with emphasis on complex carbohydrates.
- Protein intake should provide the remainder of the calories.
- Sodium intake should not exceed 3 grams per day.
- Alcohol consumption should not exceed 1 to 2 ounces of ethanol per day.
- Total calories should be sufficient to maintain the person's recommended weight.
- A wide variety of foods should be consumed.

Coffee and other caffeinated beverages should be avoided due to their ability to alter normal rate and rhythm of the heart. (2) Excessive intake of alcoholic beverages is associated with the development of heart disease due to its toxic effects to heart muscle or its association with nutritional deficiencies. (3)

NUTRIENTS

Calcium is associated with heart contraction and supplementation may increase the force of contractility in congestive heart failure. (4)

Excessive zinc and deficient copper may cause premature ventricular contraction and sudden cardiac death. (5)

In congestive heart failure there is a loss of magnesium due to activation of the renin-angiotensin-aldosterone system. Magnesium deficiency may add to the elevation of intracellular sodium and reduction of intracellular potassium, since magnesium is necessary for the Na-K pump. Supplementation with magnesium can help correct the deficiency, as well as in the correction of electrolyte imbalance involving sodium and potassium. (6) Magnesium deficiency is associated with the development of heart arrhythmias. (7) Magnesium therapy is the specific, essential treatment therapy in mitral valve prolapse and treatment can partially or totally reverse the symptoms of mitral valve prolapse in about one-third of cases. (8)

Potassium deficiency may exist despite normal blood levels and is associated with arrhythmias as well as decreased tolerance to heart medications and EKG alterations. (9) In congestive heart failure potassium losses are caused by activation of the renin-angiotensin-aldosterone system and alterations of the Na-K pump. (6) Cardiac glycosides and diuretics often exacerbate, or result in low magnesium and potassium levels, which may lead to heart arrhythmias and sudden cardiac death. (10) Magnesium and potassium are more effective when administered together when the level of either is deficient due to the inability of the heart muscle to use potassium in the absence of magnesium. (11)

Heart muscle sodium levels may be elevated while blood sodium may be deficient. Activation of the renin-angiotensin-aldosterone system causes sodium retention and magnesium and potassium losses, which leads to water retention and electrolyte imbalances. (6)

Selenium deficiency is associated with the development of alcoholic heart disease. (12)

L-carnitine is synthesized in humans from the amino acid lysine in conjunction with another amino acid, methionine. Carnitine is essential for the transport of long chain fatty acids into mitochondria within cells. Mitochondria are the dynamos within cells that are responsible for the production of energy in the form of adenosine triphosphate (ATP). Heart and skeletal muscle as well as other tissues depend on fatty acid oxidation as a source of energy and need carnitine to transport the fatty acids into the mitochondria. L-carnitine produces an anti-arrhythmic effect comparable to quinidine. L-carnitine deficiency has been associated with the development of heart disease which responded to supplementation. L-carnitine has also been used in ischemic heart disease, angina pectoris, heart attack, mitral valve prolapse and endocardial fibroelastosis. (13)

Coenzyme Q-10 or ubiquinone includes a group of fat soluble benzoquinones that are involved in mitochondrial electron transport. Coenzyme Q-10 is similar in structure to vitamin K and acts as a hydrogen receptor in the mitochondrial membrane leading to the formation of ATP. Supplementation with Coenzyme Q-10 is indicated in cardiovascular disease including angina pectoris, congestive heart failure, heart disease, mitral valve prolapse and hypertensive heart disease. (14) Coenzyme Q-10 is currently widely used in Japan, the Soviet Union and Europe. In Japan, Coenzyme Q-10 is used daily by over 6 million people in the prevention and treatment of heart disease. (15)

Taurine, like magnesium, affects the membrane excitability by normalizing potassium flux in and out of the heart muscle tissue. (16) Taurine supplementation has improved signs and symptoms of congestive heart failure. (17)

BOTANICAL MEDICINES

Hawthorn (Crataegus oxyacantha), a member of the Rose family, is a shrub or tree that grows to a height of 6 meters and is native to Europe, East Asia and eastern North America. Hawthorn has white flowers that bloom in Spring, bright red fruit containing 1 to 3 nuts and long slender thorns along its stem. Hawthorn tree has been the focus of May time rituals in England and the fruit has been used throughout Europe to make jam and wine. Hawthorn has been historically used to treat heart disorders, anemia, dyspepsia, respiratory ailments and as a diuretic and astringent in menstrual complaints. Hawthorn is a remarkable cardiovascular system tonic. (18)

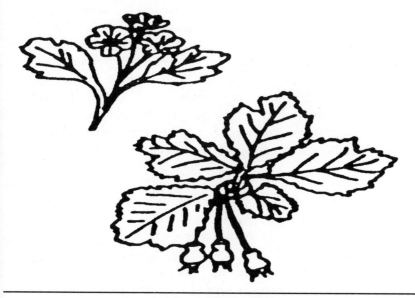

Hawthorn (Crataegus oxyacantha)

The active ingredients in Hawthorn are flavonoids. At least 30 different flavonoids have been isolated from Crataegus. The leaves, fruit, flowers and bark are all particularly high in flavonoid content. Flavonoids are responsible for imparting the color of the fruits of this plant, as well as in cherries, grapes and many other plants. The content of Hawthorn varies from 0.05 to 5.0% total flavonoid content of crude plant extract. The plant also contains tannins which are responsible for the astringent effects of Hawthorn. It should be clarified that there are variant species of Hawthorn that are of no medicinal value whatsoever. (19)

The ability of Crataegus to dilate coronary arteries and increase coronary blood flow has been widely demonstrated in both animal and human subjects. (20) Crataegus consistently increases the heart muscle contractile force as measured by amplitude of heart muscle contractility and increase in blood volume pumped. (20) Crataegus has demonstrated to decrease heart arrhythmias in Aconite induced heart rhythm disorders. (20) Variable, insignificant effects on heart rate have been observed. Crataegus has been shown to increase blood flow to skeletal muscle while at the same time decreasing blood flow to the digestive tract, kidneys and the skin. (20) Crataegus has also demonstrated to decrease blood pressure while certain flavonoids in Crataegus have been shown to increase blood pressure. (21) The duration of action is within 10 minutes following parenteral administration and after oral administration blood flow was increased over a period up to 2 hours. (22) The pharmacologic effects of Crataegus can be summarized as follows:1. An increase in coronary blood flow.2. An increase in peripheral blood flow, including skeletal muscle.3. An increase in the contractile force of heart muscle contraction.4. A decrease in heart muscle oxygen use.5. Variable, minor changes in heart rate depending on heart condition.6. A indirect decrease in blood pressure.

In Europe, over 112 products contain Crataegus and numerous standardized Hawthorn products are used in clinical medicine and available at health food stores. Crataegus is effective in improving heart condition in a number of cardiovascular disorders including congestive heart failure, angina pectoris and coronary insufficiency, arrhythmias, especially extrasystoles and paroxysmal tachycardia and heart attack. Crataegus is also indicated for high blood pressure. It dilates coronary arteries by inhibiting smooth muscle contraction, possesses mild diuretic action and has been shown to inhibit angiotensin converting enzyme (ACE) in a manner similar to many of the ACE inhibitors available from the pharmaceutical industry. (23)

The New York Heart Association stages of loss of cardiac output include 4 stages:

Stage 1. loss of capacity, means the patient is symptom free when at rest.
Stage 2. loss of capacity with medium effort and more.
Stage 3. loss of capacity with minor effort that results in obvious labored or difficult breathing.
Stage 4. patient experiences symptoms when at rest.

Crataegus is indicated in Stage 2 and 3 of the NYHA scale of loss of cardiac output. (24,25)

A study of 120 patients, designed to test the efficacy of an alcoholic extract of fruits and leaves of Crataegus monogyna and Crataegus oxyacantha was conducted in 1981. The results indicated that general condition and heart output were significantly improved, especially in regards to the associated symptoms of shortness of breath and heart palpitations. (24)

Crataegus and its extracts are non-toxic and completely safe for long term use. Few adverse side effects have been reported in over a hundred years of clinical use. Toxicity to the fetus is of little concern, since Crataegus is usually indicated for elderly patients with cardiovascular problems. (26)

RECOMMENDATIONS: Daily unless otherwise stated:

Calcium..800-1200 mg
Magnesium...400-800 mg
Potassium..2000-4000 mg
Copper...2-4 mg
Selenium...200-400 mcg
L-Carnitine...1500-3000 mg
Coenzyme Q-10..30-60 mg
Taurine...4-6 gm
Crataegus oxyacantha (4:1)......................................400-800 mg

REFERENCES

(1) Branch WT: Office Practice of Medicine. WB Saunders Company, Philadelphia, Pennsylvania, 1987

(2) Dobmeyer DJ et al: The arrhythmogenic effects of caffeine in human beings. New Engl. J. Med. 308(14):814-16, 1983

(3) Burch GE et al: Alcoholic cardiomyopathy. The Biology of Alcoholism: Vol. 3: Clinical Pathology, New York, Plenum. 1974

(4) Opie LH: Priniciples of therapy for congestive heart failure. Eur. Heart J. 4 Suppl. A:199-208, 1983

(5) Spencer JC: Direct relationship between the body's copper/zinc ratio, ventricular premature beats and sudden cardiac death. Letter to the Editor. Am. J. Clin. Nutr. June, 1979 pp 1184-5, 1983

(6) Wester PO et al: Intracellular electrolytes in cardiac failure. Acta Med. Scand. (Suppl.) 707:33-36, 1986

(7) Podell RN: The magnesium mavens: Much ado about something. Postgrad. Med. 78(5):219, 1985

(8) Durlach J et al: Latent tetany and mitral valve prolapse due to chronic primary magnesium deficit, in Halpern and Durlach, eds. Magnesium Deficiency. First European Congress in Magnesium. Karger, Basel, 1985

(9) Sangiori GB et al: Serum potassium levels, red-blood-cell potassium and alterations of the repolarization phase of electrocardiography in old subjects. Age Aging 13:309, 1984

(10) Altura BM et al: Biochemistry and pathophysiology of congestive heart failure. Is there a role for magnesium? Magnesium 5(3-4):134-43, 1986

(11) Dychner T et al: Magnesium and potassium in serum and muscle in relation to disturbances of cardiac rhythm, in Magnesium in Heart and Disease. spectrum Publishing Company, pp. 551-7, 1980

(12) Goldman IS et al: Cardiomyopathy associated with selenium deficiency. Letter to the Editor. New. Engl. J. Med. 305:701, 1982

(13) Pizzorno JE and Murray MT: Textbook of Natural Medicine. JBC Publications, Seattle, Washington, 1988(14) Gaby AR et al: Textbook of Natural Medicine. JBC Publications, Seattle, Washington, 1988

(15) Folkers K et al: Biomedical and Clinical Aspects of Coenzyme Q. Vol. 1. Elsevier/North Holland Biomedical Press, 1977

(16) Chazov EL et al: Taurine and electrical activity of the heart. Cir. Res. 34-5, Suppl. III, pp. 11-21, 1974

(17) Azume J et al: Therapeutic effect of taurine in congestive heart failure: A double-blind crossover trial. Clin. Cardiol. 8:276-82, 1985

(18) Grieve M: A Modern Herbal. Vol. 1, pp. 385-6, Dover Publications, New York, NY, 1971

(19) Wagner H et al: Cardiotonic Drugs IV, cardiotonic amines from Crataegus oxyacantha. Planta Medica 45:98-101, 1982

(20) Ammon HPT et al: Crataegus, Toxicology and Pharmacology Part II: Pharmacodynamics. Planta Medica Vol. 43 No. 3, November, 1981

(21) Petkov V: Plants with hypotensive, antiatheromatous and coronarodilating action. Am. J. Clin. Med. 7:197-236, 1979

(22) Ammon HPT et al: Crataegus, Toxicology and Pharmacology Part III: Pharmacodynamics and Pharmacocinetics. Planta Medica Vol. 43 No. 4, December 1981

(23) Uchida S et al: Inhibitory effects of condensed tannins on angiotensin converting enzyme. Jap. J. Pharmacol, 43:242-5, 1987

(24) Iwamoto M et al: Clinical effects of Crataegutt in ischaemic heart disease and/or hypertensive origin. Planta Medica Vol. 42 No. 1, 1980

(25) O'Connolly M et al: Treating older, multi-morbid patients with angina pectoris symptoms, a placebo controlled crossover double-blind study with Crataegutt novo. Therapiewoche 37:3587

(26) Ammon HPT et al: Crataegus, Toxicology and Pharmacology Part I: Toxicology. Planta Medica Vol. 43 No. 2, October 1981

CHAPTER 12

HELP FOR ARTHRITIS AND RHEUMATISM

Osteoarthritis (OA) is a non-inflammatory joint disease marked by breakdown of cartilage around bone and the build up of bone at bony margins. Osteoarthritis is the most common form of arthritis and affects approximately 20% of the general population. The incidence of osteoarthritis increases with age and tends to affect females more than males. Characteristic symptoms of osteoarthritis include joint stiffness particularly in the morning. Bone spurs and bony deformation are common in advanced cases. Rheumatoid arthritis (RA) is a chronic disease characterized by usually symmetric inflammation of the peripheral joints of the arms and legs.

About 1% of all populations are affected; women 2 to 3 times more commonly than men. Onset of rheumatoid arthritis may be abrupt, with simultaneous inflammation in multiple joints and with insidious, progressive joint involvement. Characteristic symptoms of classic rheumatoid arthritis include morning stiffness, tenderness, pain on motion, swelling and subcutaneous nodules. The exact cause of RA is still unknown. In chronically affected joints the delicate synovial membrane abnormally thickens and develops numerous folds leading to inflammation, fibrosis and necrosis. Rheumatism is the general term used to describe early arthritic changes in joints and connective tissue. Stiffness, pain and slight inflammation in joints, cartilage and other connective tissue is common.

Conventional therapy consists of analgesics, NSAID's (non-steroidal anti-inflammatory drugs), corticosteroids, immune-suppressive drugs and surgery. While conventional treatment is moderately effective, there are safe and effective natural therapies that may be effective in treating arthritis and rheumatism.

DIET

Malnutrition has been linked to arthritis and it has been suggested that malnutrition alters the way vitamins and nutrients are dealt with by the body. (1) RA patients on a low fat diet for about 1 year experienced remission of their symptoms. Most patients reported that they felt less pain and were able to function better. (2) Food sensitivities have also been implicated in the development and exacerbation of arthritis, especially rheumatoid arthritis. (3) Fasting and elimination diets may produce temporary improvement of symptoms and subsequent food challenges may produce acute exacerbations. Dairy, wheat, animal protein, food additives and preservatives have been implicated as offending agents. (4) Furthermore, hydrochloric acid deficiency has been reported in some arthritis sufferers. (5)

NUTRIENTS

Pantothenic acid (Vitamin B5) was found to be significantly deficient in many arthritis sufferers, with the degree of deficiency directly related to the severity of symptoms. (6) Supplementation in the form of calcium pantothenate produced significant improvement of the symptoms associated with arthritis. (7)

Plasma and white blood cell concentration of Vitamin C was found to be decreased in arthritic patients. (8)

Menadione (Vitamin K) is a hydrogen accepting molecule that stabilizes lysosomal membranes in the synovium and may help decrease intracellular pH of inflamed cells. (9)

Serum and synovial fluid copper concentrations are significantly elevated in patients with rheumatoid arthritis. (10) Copper concentration is directly related to the length and the severity of the disease. (11) Copper has demonstrated remarkable anti-inflammatory and analgesic effects. Copper's anti-inflammatory effect appears to be related to its ability to form complexes that serve as selective antioxidants, thus reducing localized swelling and inflammation. (12) Supplementation with copper salicylates markedly improves the symptoms of arthritic sufferers. (13) In animal models, supplementation with copper salicylate is more effective than copper or aspirin alone.

(14) Copper bracelets worn around the wrist provides a source of copper that the body absorbs and utilizes and has demonstrated to decrease swelling and inflammation. (15)

Iron levels are significantly elevated in the synovial fluid of arthritis sufferers when compared to normal individuals. (16) Iron supplementation is still however, controversial and may lead to the development of highly reactive and damaging free radicals. (17)

Total body turnover of the element manganese is lower in RA patients. (18)

Selenium is significantly decreased in arthritic sufferers when compared to normal individuals. (19)

Sulphur may be deficient and supplementation may improve arthritis symptoms. (20) Serum levels of zinc is markedly decreased while synovial fluid levels are markedly increased in RA patients. (21)

Zinc supplementation improves symptoms associated with RA including joint swelling, morning stiffness and walking time. (22)

The amino acid L-Histidine is lower in serum of RA patients and supplementation may be beneficial. (23)

Fish oil containing eicosapentaenoic acid is a rich source of Omega-3 fatty acids. Long term administration of fish oil significantly decreases pain, swelling and morning stiffness. (24) Evening primrose oil, a rich source of Omega-6 fatty acids, also produces of improvement of symptoms following administration for 4 to 12 weeks. (25)

One study showed that a combination of zinc, Vitamin C, niacin and Pyridoxine (Vitamin B6), was just as effective as conventional treatment with non-steroidal analgesics. (26)

BOTANICAL MEDICINES

Tumeric (Curcuma longa) is a perennial herb of the Ginger family that is a major ingredient of curry powder. Tumeric contains 0.3 to 5.4% of a non-volatile yellow coloring matter identified as curcumin.

Tumeric also contains 0.3 to 7.2% of an orange volatile oil. (27) Curcumin exhibits anti-inflammatory activity comparable to phenylbutazone, ibuprofen and the steroidal anti-inflammatory, cortisone. (28) Curcumin is indicated in virtually all inflammatory conditions and although its use for rheumatoid arthritis has not been clinically documented, it is indicated in this chronic inflammatory condition.

Devil's claw (Harpagophytum procumbens) is a plant indigenous to the Kalahari desert and Namibian steppes of southwest Africa. Devil's claw has been used by native Africans as a folk remedy for diseases ranging from liver and kidney disorders to allergies, headaches and most commonly, rheumatisms. (29)

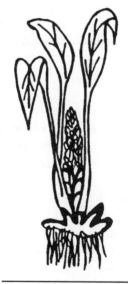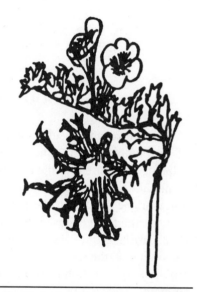

Tumeric (Curcuma longa)   Devil's claw (Harpagophytum procumbens)

The major chemical component, which has been thought to responsible for the anti-inflammatory activity of devil's claw is harpagoside. Harpagoside is primarily found in the roots of the plant ranging from 1.4 to 2.0% harpagoside. (30)

The reported anti-inflammatory activity of devil's claw remains quite controversial. Some studies indicate that devil's claw has no or only weak anti-inflammatory activity, while other studies show significant anti-inflammatory activity. When tested in animals, oral doses of the dried aqueous extracts of the root administered at 1 gram/kg had no significant effect on swelling when compared with the standard anti-inflammatory drug indomethacin. (30) In one German study, devil's claw exhibited anti-inflammatory activity comparable to phenylbutazone. (31) Analgesia was observed along with a reduction in abnormally high uric acid and cholesterol levels. In another study, 13 patients were given 410 mg of a dried aqueous extract of devil's claw three times a day over of period of six weeks, while they were continuing to take their usual anti-arthritic medications. (32) Four patients showed some subjective improvement in the symptoms. Despite the lack of documented anti-inflammatory and anti-arthritic activity in human subjects, the plant and its extracts continues to be widely used as in Europe for its anti-arthritic effects.

Harpagoside has been found to be of low toxicity. Adverse side effects in human studies include headache, tinnitus, and anorexia. (33)

FOOD SUPPLEMENTS

Glucosamine sulphate is a relatively small molecule consisting of the simple sugar, glucose, nitrogen and sulphur. Glucosamine sulphate is required for the manufacturing of joint cartilage, specifically compounds called GAG or glycosaminoglycans. Production of glucosamine appears to be the rate limiting step in the production of joint cartilage. Glucosamine sulphate becomes incorporated into the joint cartilage. Repeating units of glucosamine form the structural backbone of the glycosaminoglycans. Sulphur is important in the crosslinking of different strand of cartilage and improves the cartilage strength. The first process to occur in early arthritis is degeneration of joint cartilage. Supplementation with glucosamine sulphate helps to prevent this deterioration and actually promotes the buildup of new, healthy cartilage. (34)

Numerous double blind clinical studies show that glucosamine sulphate helps to relieve arthritic pain and inflammation. In one large double blind study involving 1,506 arthritic patients took 500 milligrams of glucosamine sulphate three times per day or placebo for an average of 50 days. 95% of patients who took glucosamine reported subjective improvement in the quality of the pain and inflammation.

(35) In another clinical study that compared glucosamine sulphate to a NSAID (non-steroidal anti-inflammatory drug) called ibuprofen, the active ingredient in Advil, Motrin or Nuprin. Pain scores decreased in the ibuprofen treated group for 2 weeks. However, by week 4 the glucosamine treated group reported better pain relief. With NSAIDs there is a growing body of evidence that while these drugs relieve pain, they actually prevent repair of joint cartilage and they promote further joint destruction. (36)

Glucosamine sulphate is very safe and non-toxic. Occasional allergic reactions, skin rash, nausea, upset stomach, heartburn and diarrhea have been reported. It is rapidly absorbed following oral consumption and localizes to connective tissue of the body including ligaments, tendons and cartilage. It is safe for long term use. It is best to take this supplement for at least 8 weeks to determine if it helps for arthritis.

RECOMMENDATIONS: Daily unless otherwise stated

Pantothenic Acid (Calcium pantothenate)..............500-1500 mg
Vitamin C..1000-5000 mg
Vitamin K...15-30 mg
Copper (Copper salicylate).................................64-128 mg
Selenium...200-400 mcg
Sulphur...500-1000 mg
Zinc...50-100 mg
Manganese..15 mg
L-Histidine...500-1000 mg
Omega-3 Oil (Max EPA)..3-6 gm
Omega-6 Oil (Evening primrose oil).............................3-6 gm
HCl supplements..3-6 caps
Curcuma longa (10:1)..50-100 mg
Harpagophytum procumbens (4:1).............................500-1500 mg
Glucosamine sulphate.......................................1000-2000 mg

REFERENCES

(1) McDuffie FC: Arthritis Foundation - reported in Med. World News, July 22, 1985
(2) Lucas C et al: Dietary fat aggravates active rheumatoid arthritis. Clin. Res.

29(4):754A, 1981

(3) Marshall R et al: Food challenge effects on fasted rheumatoid arthritis patients: A multicenter study. Clin. Ecol. 2:181-190, 1984

(4) Darlington LG et al: Placebo-controlled blind study of dietary manipulation therapy in rheumatoid arthritis. Lancet pp. 236-38, February 1, 1986

(5) Hartung EF et al: Gastric acidity in chronic arthritis. Ann. Int. Med. 9:252-7, 1935

(6) Barton-Wright EC et al: The pantothenic acid metabolism of rheumatoid arthritis. Lancet 2:862-63, 1963

(7) Calcium pantothenate in arthritic conditions. A report from the General Practitioner Research Group. Practitioner 224:208-11, 1980

(8) Mullen A et al: The metabolism of ascorbic acid in rheumatoid arthritis. Proc. Nutr. Sci. 35:8A-9A, 1976

(9) Chayen J et al: The effect of experimentally induced redox changes on human rheumatoid and non-rheumatoid synovial tissue in vitro. Beitr. Path. Bd. 149:127, 1973

(10) Niedermeier W: Concentration and chemical state of copper in synovial fluid and blood serum patients with rheumatoid arthritis. Ann. Rheum. Dis. 24:544, 1965

(11) Sorenson J: The anti-inflammatory activities of copper complexes, metal ions and biological systems. Marcel Dekker. pp. 77-125, 1982

(12) Sorenson J: Copper aspirinate: A more potent anti-inflammatory and anti-ulcer agent. J. Intern. Acad. Prev. Med. pp 7-21, 1980

(13) Sorenson RJR et al: Treatment of rheumatoid and degenerative diseases with copper complexes: A review with emphasis on copper-salicylate. Inflammation 2:217, 1977

(14) Hangarter W: Copper salicylate in rheumatoid arthritis and rheumatism-like degenerative diseases. Med. Welt. 31:1625, 1980

(15) Walker WR et al: An investigation of the therapeutic value of the "copper bracelet". Dermal assimilation of copper in arthritic/rheumatoid conditions. Agents & Actions 6:454, 1976

(16) Niedermeier W et al: Trace metal composition of synovial fluid and blood serum of patients with rheumatoid arthritis. J. Chron. Dis. 23:527-36, 1971

(17) Rawley DA et al: Formation of hydroxyl radicals from hydrogen peroxide and iron salts by superoxide and ascorbate-dependent mechanisms. Clin. Sci. 64:649-53, 1983

(18) Coltzias GC et al: Slow turnover of manganese in active rheumatoid arthritis and acceleration by prednisone. J Clin. Invest. 47:992, 1968

(19) Jahansson V et al: Nutritional status in girls with juvenile chronic arthritis. Human Nutr. Clin. Nutr. 40C:57-67, 1986

(20) Sullivan MX et al: Cystine content of finger nails in arthritis. J. Bone & Joint Surg. 16:185, 1935

(21) Niedermeier W et al: Trace metal composition of synovial fluid and blood serum of patients with rheumatoid arthritis. J. Chron. Dis. 23:527-36, 1971

(22) Simkin PA: Oral zinc sulphate in rheumatoid arthritis. Lancet 2:539, 1976

(23) Pinals RS et al: Treatment of rheumatoid arthritis with L-Histidine. J. Rheumatol. 4(4):414-419, 1977

(24) Kremer JM et al: effect of manipulation of dietary fatty acids on clinical manifestations of rheumatoid arthritis. Lancet 1:184-7, 1985

(25) Horribin DF: The importance of gamma-linolenic acid and prostaglanding E1 in human nutrition and medicine. J. Holistic Med. 3:118-139, 1981

(26) Hansen TM et al: Treatment of rheumatoid arthritis with prostaglandin E1 precursors cis-linoleic acid and gamma-linolenic acid. Scand. J. Rheum. 12:85, 1983

(27) Leung AY: Encyclopedia of Common Natural Ingredients Used in Food, Drugs, and Cosmetics. John Wiley & Sons, 1980

(28) Mukhopadhyay A et al: Antiinflammatory and irritant activities of curcumin analogues in rats. Agents Actions 12:508-515, 1982

(29) Duke JA: Handbook of Medicinal Herbs. CRC Press, Boca Raton, FL, 1985

(30) The Lawrence Review of Natural Products: Devil's Claw. Pharmaceutical Information Associates, Ltd., Levittown, Pennsylvania, July 1987

(31) Kampf R. Schweiz Apothek Zeitung 114:337, 1976

(32) Graham R et al: : Ann. Rheum. Dis. 40:632, 1981

(33) Whitehouse LW et al: Devil's claw (Harpagophytum procumbens): no evidence for anti-inflammatory activity in the treatment of arthritic disease. Canadian Med. Assoc. J. 129:249-51, 1983

(34) Murray MT: Glucosamine sulfate: Effective osteoarthritis treatment. Am. J. Nat. Med. pp.10-14, September, 1994

(35) Tapadinhas MJ et al: Oral glucosamine sulfate in the management of arthrosis: report on multi-centre open investigation in Portugal. Pharmatherapeutica 3:157-68, 1982

(36) Vaz AL: double-blind clinical evaluation of the relative efficacy of ibuprofen and glucosamine in outpatients with gonarthrosis. Clin. Ther. 3:336-43, 1982

CHAPTER 13

IMPROVING EYESIGHT AND VISION

The macule is the central area of the retina in the eye responsible for fine vision. Macular degeneration is the leading cause of decreased visual acuity in people aged 55 or older in North America and is second only to cataracts as the leading cause of decreased vision in people aged 65 or older. Macular degeneration is responsible for blindness in approximately 120,000 people in North America and accounts for 16,000 new cases of blindness each year. Risk factors to the development of macular degeneration include atherosclerosis and hypertension. There is no effective conventional medical treatment for macular degeneration. Natural therapies exist that help prevent macular degeneration.

NUTRIENTS

Nutritional antioxidants including vitamin A, vitamin C, vitamin E and Selenium protect cell membranes from the damaging effects of free radicals that is associated with macular degeneration. (1)

Zinc supplementation prevents accelerated visual loss that is associated with macular degeneration. In one clinical study involving 151 patients, those patients who received 200 mg of zinc sulphate had significantly less visual loss than the placebo group. (2)

BOTANICAL MEDICINES

Ginkgo biloba has been widely used to treat vascular insufficiency problems in the brain and extremities. Ginkgo has been used to treat patients suffering from macular degeneration. In one clinical study of ten patients with macular degeneration, a statistically significant improvement in long term visual acuity was observed after treatment with Ginkgo biloba extract. (3)

Bilberry (Vaccinium myrtillus), native to northern Europe and Asia, is a cousin to the North American blueberry and huckleberry. Bilberry has been used to make jam for hundreds of years. Medicinal use of bilberry became popular during World War II when British RAF pilots consumed bilberries prior to night flying. They believed that consumption of bilberries significantly improved their night vision during their missions. (4)

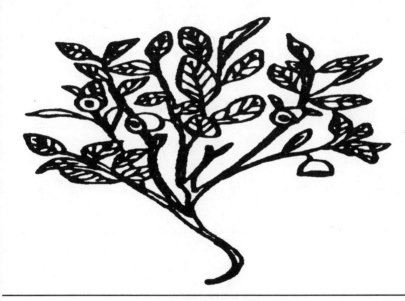

Bilberry (Vaccinium myrtillus)

The active constituents of bilberry are anthocyanosides. In fresh fruit the anthocyanidin content is approximately 0.1 to 0.25% of the crude weight of the berries. Concentrated Bilberry extracts are standardized to contain 20 to 25% anthocyanoside content. (5)

Bilberry anthocyanosides stabilize connective tissue by increasing the integrity of the collagen matrix, increasing the synthesis of collagen and preventing destruction of the collagen connective tissue around blood vessels. (6) Anthocyanosides are also potent antioxidants which prevent cell membrane damage from free radicals. (7) Bilberry anthocyanosides decrease capillary fragility and permeability which prevents inflammation. (8) Bilberry anthocyanosides have also demonstrated vascular smooth muscle relaxing effects and significantly inhibit platelet aggregation. (9) Anthocyanosides also speed up regeneration of rhodopsin, a visual pigment in the retina of the eye responsible, in part, for the conversion of light into electrical energy. Anthocyanosides stimulate dark adaption and improvement of visual acuity in normal adults. (10)

Bilberry has been effectively used in the treatment of a variety of visual problems including night blindness, visual fatigue from eye strain, diabetic retinopathy, cataracts and macular degeneration. (11)

Bilberry is virtually non-toxic and few adverse side effects have been reported. Doses of up to 400 mg/kg have been administered to rats without any apparent side effects. (12,13)

RECOMMENDATIONS: Daily unless otherwise stated

Vitamin A..10,000 IU
Vitamin C...200 mg
Vitamin E...400 IU
Selenium..400 mcg
Zinc..50 mg
Ginkgo biloba (4:1)..120 mg
Vaccinium myrtillus (4:1)...100 mg

REFERENCES

(1) Pizzorno JE and Murray MT: A Textbook of Natural Medicine. JBC Publications, Seattle, Wash. 1986

(2) Newsome DA et al: Oral zinc in macular degeneration. Arch. Ophthalmol. 106:192-8, 1988

(3) Lebuisson DA et al: Treatment of senile macular degeneration with ginkgo biloba extract. A preliminary double-blind, drug versus placebo study. Press Med. 15:1556-8. 1986

(4) Grieve M: A Modern Herbal, volume 1. Dover Publications, New York, NY, 1971

(5) Baj A et al: Qualitative and quantitative evaluation of Vaccinium myrtillus anthocyanins by high-resolution gas chromatography and high performance liquid chromatography. J. Chromatogr. 270: 279:365-72, 1983

(6) Gabor M: Pharmacologic effects of flavonoids on blood vessels. Angiologica 9:355-

74, 1972

(7) Monboisse JC et al: Oxygen-free radical as mediators of collagen breakage. Agents Actions 15:49-50, 1984

(8) Kuhnau J: The Flavonoids: A class of semi-essential food components: Their role in human nutrition. Wld. Rev. Nutr. Diet 24:117-91, 1976

(9) Rasmussen C: Anthocyanosides. Adhesivite plaqyettaire et prevention des thromboses. Therapeutique 48:399, 1972

(10) Alfieri R et al: Influence des anthocyanosides administres par voie parenterale sur l'adaptoelectroretinogramme du lapin. C.R. Soc. Biol. 158:2338, 1964

(11) Mowrey, DB: Next Generation Herbal Medicine. Comorant Books, Lehi, Utah, 1988

(12) Leitti A and Forni G: Studies on Vaccinium myrtillus anthocyanosides I. Vasoprotective and anti-inflammatory activity. Arzneim. Forsch. 26:829-32, 1976

(13) Leitti A and Forni G: Studies on Vaccinium myrtillus anthocyanosides II. Aspects of anthocyanins pharmacokinetics in the rat. Arzneim. Forsch. 26:832-5, 1976

CHAPTER 14

NATURAL PAIN RELIEF

Pain is a more or less localized sensation of discomfort, distress or agony resulting from the stimulation of specialized nerve endings throughout the body. Pain of varying degrees is a common and for the most part unpleasant sensation to all of us. Conventional pharmacologic control of pain involves the use of Aspirin (Acetylsalicylic acid) and Acetaminophen. While these drugs are effective for mild to moderate pain relief they are not without adverse side effects. The main adverse side effects to aspirin use is stomach intolerance. Aspirin irritates and erodes the protective lining of the stomach and may lead to the development of stomach ulcers. With higher doses of aspirin, patients may experience decreased hearing, vertigo (spinning sensation) and tinnitus (ringing in the ears). In addition, aspirin may cause mild, usually asymptomatic hepatitis and is associated with the development of Reye's syndrome. Reye's syndrome is occasionally seen in children under 18 years following a viral infection and is characterized by inflammation of the brain and fatty degeneration of the liver. Acetaminophen is associated with the development of liver damage. Natural substitutes exist that are effective for the control of mild to moderate pain and don't have the serious side effects of conventional medications.

DIET

Coffee and other caffeine containing products decrease the effectiveness of painkillers. Coffee has a powerful opiate receptor binding capacity that antagonizes the the analgesic effects of the body's natural pain killer's, endorphins and enkephalins. Increase consumption of hot and spicy foods, including cayenne, tumeric and ginger, if tolerated. These foods contain natural pain relieving chemicals. (1)

NUTRIENTS

The amino acid phenylalanine has shown to be effective for chronic pain relief even when standard medications have provided limited or no relief. (2) Phenylalanine appears to inhibit the enzymes involved in enkephalin degradation and thereby increases the levels of these naturally occuring painkillers. (3) Phenylalanine supplementation provided good relief for chronic pain in individuals with post-surgical low back pain, osteoarthritis, whiplash, rheumatoid arthritis, fibrositis and migraine headaches. (4)

L-Tryptophan is an amino acid precursor to the brain neurotransmitter serotonin, which is involved in pain tolerance. Tryptophan has mild analgesic action similar to aspirin and acetaminophen. (5) L-Tryptophan supplementation increases the pain tolerance threshold and reverses tolerance developed to opiates. (6) Tryptophan has provided effective pain relief for patients suffering from dental, facial and headache pain. (7)

BOTANICAL MEDICINES

White Willow bark (Salix alba) and related species are a major source of natural salicylates. Willow bark does not contain salicylic acids like aspirin, but rather the glycoside salicin, at quite high levels ranging from 2.0 to 7.0% of the crude weight of the plant.

Willow bark has been used medicinally for centuries to treat rheumatoid arthritis, connective tissue inflammation and fevers. White willow bark has been used by the Egyptians, Assyrians and Greeks and has been mentioned in manuscripts by Galen, Hippocrates and Dioscorides.

In 1829, salicin was isolated from willow bark and in 1838, salicin was converted to salicylic acid. In 1853, salicylic acid was converted to acetylsalicylic acid and aspirin was created. White willow bark, though effective, was replaced by widespread use of aspirin for analgesia by the turn of century. White willow bark remains as a high source of natural salicylates that is effective in treating mild to moderate pain. (8)

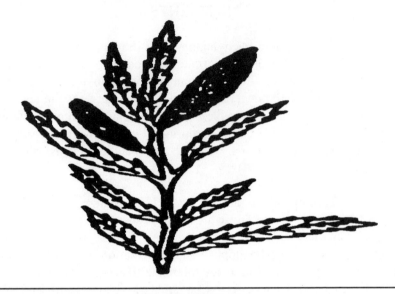

White Willow (Salix alba)

RECOMMENDATIONS: Daily unless otherwise stated

DL-Phenylalanine..1-2 gm
Salix alba (8:1)..1000-2000 mg

REFERENCES

(1) Boublik JH et al: Coffee contains potent opiate receptor binding activity. Nature 301:246-48, 1983
(2) Balagot R et al. Adv. Pain Res. Ther. 5:289-292, 1983
(3) Budd K: Use of D-phenylalanine, an enkephalinase inhibitor, in the treatment of intractable pain. Adv. Pain Res. & Therapy 5:305-308, 1983
(4) Ehhrenpreis S et al: Naloxone reversible analgesia in mice produced by D-phenylalanine and hydrocinnamic acid, inhibitors of carboxypepitase A. Adv. Pain Res & Therapy, Vol. 3, 1978
(5) Liberman Hr et al: Mood, performance and pain sensitivity: Changes induced by food constituents. J. Psychiat. Res. 17:181-6, 1982-3
(6) Seltzer S et al: Alteration of human pain thresholds by nutritional manipulation and L-Tryptophan supplementation. Pain 13(4):385-93, 1982
(7) Seltzer S et al: Perspectives in the control of chronic pain by nutritional manipulation. Pain 11(2):121-48, 1981
(8) Duke JA: Handbook of Medicinal Herbs. CRC Press, Boca Raton, FL., 1985

CHAPTER 15

PRESCRIPTION FOR DEPRESSION

Depression, the most common psychological disturbance in the general population, is a disturbance characterized by depression with or without anxiety. Ten to 20% of the general population, 20 to 50% of patients seen in general practice settings, to 30 to 60% of general hospital inpatients suffer from depression. Depression is characterized by poor appetite with weight loss or increased appetite with weight gain, insomnia or hypersomnia, psychomotor agitation or retardation, loss of interest or pleasure in usual activities or decrease in sexual drive, loss of energy and feelings of fatigue, feelings of worthlessness, self-reproach, or inappropriate guilt, diminished ability to think and concentrate, recurrent thoughts of suicide or death. There are two major categories of depression. In unipolar depression there is one or more episodes of depression alone, while in bipolar depression the episodes of depression are alternated with episodes of mania. Undiagnosed medical illness often presents as depression and should be considered in the evaluation of any depressed patient. Hormone dysfunction, infectious disease and cancer, most notably pancreatic cancer, present with the symptom of depression. Five percent of depressed patients have a specific psychological disorder that is known to respond to medication. Commonly used medication include propranolol, methyldopa, reserpine, anti-anxiety drugs and corticosteroids. Safe and effective natural alternatives exist for the treatment of depression and should be considered.

NUTRIENTS

Biotin deficiency may cause depression as part of a syndrome including headaches, nausea, insomnia, lethargy and muscle weakness and supplementation alleviates the symptoms. (1)

Folic acid deficiency is associated with the development of depression and supplementation significantly reduces the incidence of depression. (2)

Pyridoxine (Vitamin B6) is an important coenzyme required in the production of monoamine neurotransmitters in the brain. The use of monoamine oxidase inhibitors (MAOI) may cause deficiency of pyridoxine and result in depression. Pyridoxine is necessary for the conversion of tryptophan into the neurotransmitter serotonin, which when deficient may cause depression. The use of estrogen and progesterone hormones, as with oral contraceptives, is associated with increased urinary excretion of tryptophan metabolites, as happens with pyridoxine deficiency. Disturbances of tryptophan metabolism have been shown to be responsible for depression, anxiety, decrease in libido and impairment of glucose tolerance. Supplementation with pyridoxine corrects the deficiency and alleviates the symptoms associated with the deficiency. (3)

Riboflavin (Vitamin B2) deficiency is associated with the development of depression. (4)

Thiamine (Vitamin B1) deficiency is marked by the development of depression and irritability. (5)

Vitamin B12 deficiency may cause depression, even in the absence of anemia. (6)

Impaired Vitamin C levels may result in chronic depression, tiredness, irritability and general ill-health. (7)

Calcium supplementation may be especially effective for post-menopausal and post-delivery depression and depression among the elderly. (8)

Chronic iron deficiency, most commonly associated in women with menstrual problems, is associated with a marked depression of monamine oxidase activity and development of depression. (9)

Magnesium deficiency is associated with development of depression and may be necessary in maintaining normal serotonin levels in cerebrospinal fluid. (10)

Potassium deficiency is frequently associated with a dysphoric mood, tearfulness, weakness and fatigue. Depressed patients may have decreased intracellular potassium levels despite normal blood levels. (11)

Vanadium has shown to be a powerful inhibitor of Na/K ATPase activity and is associated with the development of melancholia and depression. (12)

Evening primrose oil is a high source of gamma linoleic acid (GLA), a precursor to prostaglandin E1, which may be deficient in patients with depression. (13)

The amino acid, L-Phenylalanine is a precursor to L-Tyrosine, which is a precursor to the brain neurotransmitter, dopamine. (14) L-Phenylalanine can be converted to phenylethylamine (PEA), an amphetamine-like neurotransmitter which is found in high quantities in chocolate and has been shown to have stimulatory properties. (15) Supplementation with L-Phenylalanine may benefit depressed patients.

The amino acid, L-Tryptophan a precursor to the brain neurotransmitter serotonin, may be deficient in patients with depression and supplementation may be beneficial. (16) Deficiency of the amino acid L-Tyrosine, a precursor to the brain neurotransmitter dopamine, may benefit patients suffering from depression. (17) Supplementation with L-Tryptophan and L-Tyrosine may be an effective treatment of depression because it enhances both serotonin and catecholamine metabolism. (18)

OTHER FACTORS

Food sensitivities may cause mental and behavioral symptoms by a variety of mechanisms including cerebral allergy, food addiction, hypoglycemia, caffeinism, hypersensitivity to chemical food additives, reactions to vasoactive amines in foods and reactions to neuropeptides formed from certain foods. Sugar addiction can induce dysglycemia and episodes of low blood sugar that can alter behavior. Excess consumption of caffeine beverages can alter mood and behavior. Common food allergies include dairy, wheat, chocolate, yeast, corn and a variety of food preservatives and colourings. (19)

BOTANICAL MEDICINES

St. John`s Wort (Hypericum perforatum) is a woody perennial plant that is native to Europe, Asia, Africa and is naturalized to many other parts of the world including North America and Australia. St. John`s Wort is especially prevalent in northern California and southern Oregon. The plant's common name, St. John`s Wort, is in reference to the biblical apostle St. John. Early christians believed that red spots appeared on the leaves of this plant on the exact date of the saint's beheading and so named the plant in commemoration of the saint. Hypericum has been historically used by the Greeks to treat a variety of illness including infections, wounds, respiratory problems, kidney dysfunction and depression

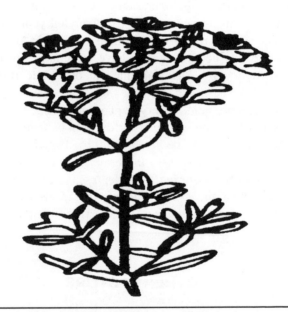

St. John's Wort (Hypericum perforatum)

The chemical composition of Hypericum is exceedingly complex.The dianthrone derivatives, hypericin and pseudohypericin, range in concentration from 0.0095 to 0.466% have demonstrated antidepressive activity. (20)

One of the current theories of depression hypothesizes that depression is a result of deficiency or decreased effectiveness of norepinephrine and serotonin acting on nerve impulse transmitting substances called neurotransmitters in the brain and central nervous system (CNS). One of the most popular methods of treating depression is with monoamine oxidase inhibitors (MAOI), which retard the major enzyme responsible for the breakdown of various neurotransmitters in the brain, thus increasing the concentration of these neurotransmitters in the brain and CNS. Extracts from Hypericum have demonstrated to inhibit both type A and B monoamine oxidase and thereby increase the levels of these neurotransmitters in the brain and CNS in a manner similar to conventional MAO inhibitors. In addition, Hypericum has demonstrated antiviral activity including the AIDS virus. Researchers from the New York University Medical center and the Weismann Institute of Science demonstrated that compounds from this plant, primarily hypericin and pseudohypericin, strongly inhibit a variety of in experimental laboratory animals. Although encouraging, the use of Hypericum in treating retroviral infections including AIDS, requires more research before its use is proven in this respect. Extracts of Hypericum have also demonstrated anti-bacterial and wound healing activity. (20)

In modern European medicine, St. John's Word extracts are included in many over-the-counter (OTC) and prescription drugs for mild depression. Other preparations are used for bedwetting and nightmares in children, gastritis and the oil is used extensively in burn and wound remedies externally. (21) A clinical study of 15 women who were treated with a standardized hypericin extract demonstrated improvement in the symptoms of depression including anxiety, dysphoric mood, hypersomnia, anorexia, motor retardation and feelings of worthlessness. In another clinical study with 6 depressed women 55 to 65 years old, administration of a standardized hypericum extract resulted in a significant increase urinary output of a chemical marker for the beginning of the antidepressive reaction. (22)

Excessive consumption of St. John's Wort in grazing animals, particularly horses, sheep, goats and cattle has resulted in photo-toxicity. The compound hypericum is absorbed from the intestine and concentrates near the skin. When the animal is exposed to sunlight an allergic reaction takes place leading to hemolysis and tissue damage. There is no evidence that this is true for humans and St. John's Wort has been consumed without side effects in doses prescribed. Exposure to excessive sunlight is discouraged while taking Hypericum extracts. (20)

RECOMMENDATIONS: Daily unless otherwise stated

Biotin...200-400 mcg
Folic Acid...400 mcg
Pyridoxine...100-200 mg
Thiamine..10-20 mg
Vitamin B12..100-1000 mcg
Vitamin C..1000-2000 mg
Calcium...1000-1500 mg
Iron..10-25 mg
Magnesium..800-1000 mg
Potassium..2000-5000 mg
Omega-6 Oil..3000 mg
DL-Phenylalanine.......................................500 mg
L-Tyrosine...4000-6000 mg
HCl..3-6 caps
Hypericum perforatum (4:1)........................1500-3000 mg

REFERENCES

(1) Levenson JL: J. Parenteral & Enteral Nutr. 7(2):181-3, 1983
(2) Ghadoroam AM et al: Folic acid deficiency and depression. Psychosomatics 2(11):926-9, 1980
(3) Bermond P: Therapy of side effects of oral contraceptive agents with vitamin B6. Acta Vitaminol. Enzymol. 4(1-2):45-54, 1982
4) Carney MW et al: Thiamine, riboflavin and pyridoxine deficiency in psychiatric in-patients. Br.J. Psychiat. 141-271-272, 1982
(5) Brozek J: Psycholocis effects of thiamine restriction and deprivation in normal young men. Am. J. Clin. Nutr. 5(2):109-20, 1957
(6) Zucker DK et al: B12 deficiency and psychiatric disorders. Biol. Psychiat. 16:197-205, 1981
(7) Schorah CJ et al: Human Nutr: Clin. Nutr. 37C:447-452, 1983
(8) Crammer J: Lithium, calcium, and mental illness. Lancet 1:215-16, 1956
(9) Parker SD: Depression and nutrition: Anemia and glucose imbalance. Anabolism Jan.-Feb., 1984
(10) Banki CM et al: Cerebrospinal fluid magnesium and calcium related to amine metabolites, diagnosis, and suicide attempts. Biol Psychiat. 20:163-171, 1985
(11) Webb WL et al: Electrolyte and fluid imbalance: Neuropsychiatric manifestations. Psychosomatics 22(3):199-203, 1981
(12) Canley LC et al: Vanadate is a potent (Na,K)-ATPase inhibitor found in ATP derived from muscle. J. Biol. Chem. 252:7421-3, 1977
(13) Lieb J et al: Prostagl. Leukotrienes & Med. 10:361-7, 1983

(14) Beckmann H: Phenylalanaine in affective disorders. Adv. Biol. Psychiat. 10:137-47, 1983

(15) Sabelli HC et al: Clinical studies on the phenylethylamine hypothesis of affective disorder. J. Clin. Psychiat. 47(2):66-70, 1986

(16) Branchey L et al: Relationship between changes in plasma amino acids and depression in alcoholic patients. Am. J. Psyychiat. 141:1212-1215, 1984

(17) Gibson CJ et al: Tyrosine for treatment of depression. Adv. Biol Psychiat. 10:148-159, 1983

(18) van Praag HM: Studies in the mechanism of action of serotonin precursors in depression. Psychopharm. Bull. 20(3):599-602, 1984

(19) Rippere V: Some varieties of food intolerance in psychiatric patients. Nutr. Health 3(3):125-36, 1984

(20) Hobbs C: St. John's Wort, Hypericum perforatum L. Herbal/Gram. 18/19:24-33, 1989

(21) Weiss RF: Herbal Medicine, Beaconsfield Publishers Ltd. Beaconsfield, England

(22) Muldner Von H et al: Antidepressive wirkung eines auf den wirkstoffkomplex hypericin standardisierten hypericum-extraktes. Arzneim-Forsch. 34:918, 1984

CHAPTER 16

PREVENTING MIGRAINE HEADACHES

A migraine, usually a severe headache, is often limited to one side of the head and is sometimes accompanied by nausea and vomiting. Stress is the single most common precipitant of migraine attacks. Other common precipitants include dietary factors, hormonal changes and hypoglycemia. A conservative estimate indicates that 10% of the North American population or ten to twenty million people suffer from migraine attacks. Up to 70% of migraine patients have a family history for migraine, suggesting a possible genetic link. Certain foods have been described to provoke attacks. Cheese, pickled herring, red wine and chocolate are all believed to provoke migraine attacks. Some individuals afflicted with migraines may have disordered carbohydrate metabolism and notice that missing a meal brings on an attack and they should eat regular, small meals. Stress reduction techniques such as meditation, hypnotherapy, acupuncture and hydrotherapy may be helpful and may provide relief. Safe and natural alternatives are available for the treatment of migraine headache.

DIET

Caffeine intake has been correlated with increased headache prevalence. (1) Caffeine withdrawal headache begins about 18 hours after caffeine ingestion and quickly develops into a diffuse, throbbing and painful headache that is exacerbated with exercise. (2)   Food sensitivities have also been implicated as a trigger of migraines. At least 25 different syndromes have been described in which foods or food and drug combinations cause head and neck pain including coloring and flavoring agents, alcoholic products, chocolate, tea, foods containing tyramine, vitamins, minerals, pesticides and other food additives and preservatives. (3) Identification and elimination of foods from the diet that provoke migraine attacks is effective in reducing the incidence of attacks. (4)

Intake of foods high in dietary copper such as chocolate or which increase intestinal absorption of copper, such as citrus fruits, potentiate headache triggering agents. The role of copper in metabolism of vasoactive amines such as serotonin, tyramine and catecholamines has been implicated as the triggering mechanism. (5)

NUTRIENTS

Supplementation with Omega-3 oils may be beneficial. (6) Omega-3 oils changes the balance of prostaglandins and leukotrienes in the body. Both prostaglandins and leukotrienes are important and powerful chemicals in the body that mediate inflammation and the immune response. Supplementation with Omega-3 oils decreases the frequency and the intensity of migraine attacks. In one clinical study of 8 migraine patients who received either 15 grams of EPA (Omega-3 oil) or placebo for six weeks, EPA reduced the incidence of severe headaches by more than half. (7)

Choline supplementation may be helpful. Red blood cell choline concentrations are lower in patients during and between cluster headaches, suggesting that addition of choline is beneficial in restoring normal choline levels. (8)

BOTANICAL MEDICINES

Feverfew (Tanacetum parthenium) is a short perennial that grows along fields and roadsides throughout North America and Europe. Feverfew, as its name suggests, has been used traditionally as an antipyretic to lower body temperature in fevers. Feverfew has been used to treat headaches, arthritis, asthma and menstrual disorders. According to legend, the ancient Greeks called feverfew "parthenium" because it was used to save the life of someone who had fallen from the Parthenon, the Doric Greek temple in Athens. Research confirms the clinical use of feverfew to treat migraine headaches. (9)

The active ingredient in feverfew is a group of compounds known as sesquiterpene lactones, the most common lactone of which, is called parthenolide. The parthenolide content of crude feverfew leaves ranges from 0.1 to 0.5% with 0.2% parthenolide content being about average. In addition the plant contains a small amount of essential oils including camphor, which partially accounts for the characteristic odor of the plant. (10)

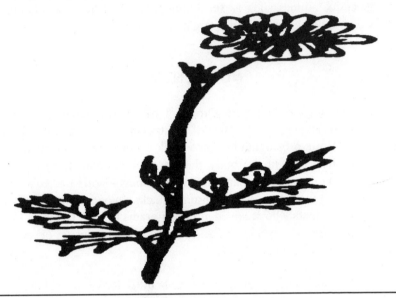

Feverfew (Tanacetum parthenium)

Active ingredients in feverfew, namely the parthenolides, have been shown to consistently inhibit platelet aggregation and secretion of the vasoactive prostaglandins and thromboxanes. Platelets are small disc-like or platelet structures that circulate in the blood and are responsible for blood clotting and coagulation. Platelets contain many active chemicals that affect the circulation of blood. Unlike aspirins that contain salicylates which blocks enzymatic pathways, feverfew directly inhibits platelet aggregation and inhibits platelets from releasing prostaglandins and thromboxanes. Feverfew interferes with the initial step of the inflammatory pathway by blocking the release of arachidonic acid from platelets and white blood cells. (11, 12) In addition, feverfew has shown antibacterial activity against gram positive bacteria, toxicity against human tumor cells and antithrombotic potential against heart attacks. (9)

A study of 270 patients who used feverfew for several months indicated that fevefew decreased both the frequency and the severity of migraine attacks. (13) In one study of 17 migraine patients who received either 50 mg of encapsulated feverfew leaf or placebo, the incidence of headache was markedly lower in the feverfew treated group as well as the incidence of nausea and vomiting. In 8 patients who received feverfew versus 9 patients who received placebo, it was concluded that feverfew users had a statistically lower number of headaches as compared to the placebo treated group. (14) In another study, 72 volunteers with a history of migraine received feverfew or placebo. The results indicated that feverfew reduced the number and severity of migraine attacks significantly. (15) Feverfew has proven to be effective in reducing both the frequency and severity of migraine headaches.

Minor and infrequent adverse reactions to feverfew have been described. The most common reaction reported by 6.7% of 270 regular users of feverfew leaf was mouth and tongue irritation and inflammation. Other reactions described include abdominal pain, indigestion, unpleasant taste, tingling, urinary problems, headache, swollen lips and mouth and diarrhea. Rapid heart rate has also been described by few patients, while nausea, insomnia and joint pain have been described by users who discontinued use of feverfew. Feverfew use during pregnancy is discouraged. (16)

RECOMMENDATIONS: Daily unless otherwise stated

Omega-3 Oil..5-10 gm
Tanacetum parthenium (4:1)....................................50 mg

REFERENCES

(1) Shirlow MJ et al: A study of caffeine consumption and symptoms: Indigestion, palpitations, tremor, headache and insomnia. Int J. Epidemiol. 14 (2):239-48, 1985(2) Greden JF et al: Caffeine withdrawal headache: A clinical profile. Psychosomatics 21:411-18, 1980
(3) Selzer S: Foods amd food and drug combinations, responsible for head and neck pain. Cephalgia 2(2):111-124, 1982
(4) O'Banion DR: Dietary control of headach pain: Five case studies. J. Holistic Med. 3:149-151, 1981
(5) Hanson DP: Copper as a factor in the dietary precipitation of migraine. Headache 26(5):248-50, 1986
(6) Mc Carren T et al: Am. J. Clin. Nutr. 41:874a, 1985

(7) Glueck C: University of Cincinnati College of Medicine. 1986

(8) de Belleroche J et al: Erythrocyte choline concentrations and cluster headache. Brt. Med J. 288:268-70, 1984

(9) Hobbs C: Feverfew, Tanacetum parthenium. Herbal/Gram 20:26-47, Spring 1989

(10) Awang DVC: Letter to the Editor. Herbal/Gram 22:2,34,42, Spring 1990

(11) Makheja AN et al: The Active Principle in Feverfew. Lancet Vol. 2, November 7, 1981

(12) Heptinstall S et al: Extracts of feverfew inhibit granule secretion in blood platelets and polymorphonuclear leukocytes. Lancet Vol. 1, May 11, 1985

(13) Mahaja AN et al: A platelet phospholipase inhibitor from the medicinal herb feverfew (Tanacetum parthenium). Prostaglandins, Leukotrienes & Med. 8:653-60, 1982

(14) Johnson ES et al: Efficacy of feverfew as prophylactic treatment of migraine. Brit. Med J. 2911: 569-73, 1985

(15) Murphy JJ et al: Randomized double-blind placebo-controlled trial of feverfew in migraine prevention. Lancet 189: July 23, 1988

(16) The Lawrence Review of Natural Products: Feverfew. Levittown, Penn. August 1986

CHAPTER 17

PREVENTING STROKES

The term cerebrovascular disease refers to any disease involving one or more of the blood vessels of the brain. A stroke or cerebrovascular accident (CVA) is a severe complication of cerebrovascular disease. A stroke involves rupture or blockage of a blood vessel in the brain, depriving parts of the brain of blood supply, resulting in loss of consciousness, paralysis, or other symptoms depending on the site and extent of brain damage. Cerebrovascular disease is a major cause of disability and the third leading cause of death in western society. The impact on society is far-reaching with an estimated annual cost greater than 7.5 billion dollars in the Unites States and Canada. Seventy-five percent of all strokes occur in individuals who are 65 years old or older. Although injury to the brain can occur as part of a number of relatively rare diseases, most cerebrovascular diseases are secondary to atherosclerotic disease, hypertension or a combination of both. Increased age, especially greater than 65, is a risk factor for the development of a stroke. Patients who suffer one stroke are at high risk for having another stroke. Cerebrovascular disease is a disease of modern society which is complicated by hypertension and atherosclerosis. There are effective, safe and non-toxic natural therapies that can play a role in preventing the development of cerebrovascular disease and its complications.

DIET

A diet high in fruit and vegetable consumption was associated with a lower incidence of cerebrovascular disease. (1) Regular alcohol consumption is associated with increased risk of cerebral hemorrhage. (2) Excessive alcohol intake may cause an acute stroke. (3) Alcohol, when consumed with a high fat meal especially saturated fats, reduces platelet aggregation and increases the chance of cerebral hemorrhage. (4) A diet high in fats and refined carbohydrates, together with a sedentary lifestyle, plays an important role in the development of atherosclerosis and hypertension.

NUTRIENTS

In experimental research vitamin E supplementation normalized platelet survival time and decreased the incidence of cerebral atherosclerosis. (5) Supplementation with Omega-3 oils, may protect against decreases in cerebral blood flow and brain swelling. (6)

BOTANICAL MEDICINES

Ginkgo biloba (Ginkgo) ,a living fossil, is considered to be the world's oldest living tree and its history can be traced back more than 200 million years. Ginkgo once grew extensively throughout Europe and North America, but now only grows in parts of China and Japan. The medicinal use of Ginkgo leaves dates to 2800 BC. The first recorded use of Ginkgo was in the Chinese Materia Medica where Ginkgo was used to improve brain function including dementia and senility, respiratory ailments and vascular problems. Individual trees grow up to 50 meters in height and may live as long as 2000 years. (7)

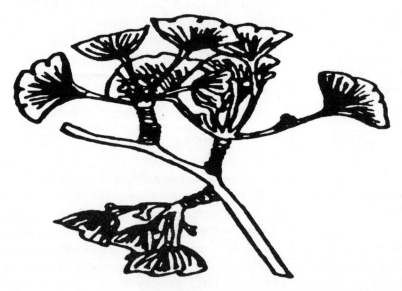

Ginkgo (Ginkgo biloba)

The pharmacologic activity of Ginkgo leaf is related to its high content of terpenes, flavonoids, proanthocyanidins and flavoglycosides (Ginkgo heterosides). Ginkgo biloba extract contains up to 24% flavoglycosides and is a widely available medicinal product throughtout Europe. (8)

Ginkgo biloba extract has been used to treat arterial insufficiency with impressive results. Ginkgo has demonstrated inhibition of platelet aggregation and subsequently, decreases the growth of atherosclerotic plaques. (9) Ginkgo stabilizes membranes involved in the blood-brain barrier.The net effect is a marked reduction in brain swelling. (10) Ginkgo flavonoids have also demonstrated antioxidant activity by binding oxygen free radicals and inhibiting membrane damage. (11) Ginkgo stimulates the synthesis of prostanoids and related substances that are capable of dilating blood vessels. (12) Ginkgo increases cerebral blood flow and decreases blood pressure. Ginkgo has also demonstrated to decrease the onset and severity of visual impairment caused by diabetes, probably due its antioxidant effects and its ability to dilate blood vessels. (13) Ginkgo has been shown to increase the synthesis of the brain neurotransmitter dopamine, which is postulated to enhance function in the brain. Ginkgo biloba extract (GBE) has also demonstrated to enhance the release of catecholamines including adrenaline and noradrenaline. Catecholamines have strong effects on both nerve and heart function. Ginkgo biloba reinforces the regulation of the sympathetic nervous system directly by acting on neuromediator release and indirectly by inhibiting their degradation by inhibiting the enzyme catechol-orthomethyltransferase. (14) In arterial walls GBE stimulates the release of endogenous relaxing factors such as endothelium derived relaxing factor and prostacyclin. (15) The action of GBE in the venous system has been shown to have a blood vessel constrictor component that maintains the degree of tone, essential to the dynamic clearing of toxic metabolites accumulated during periods of decreased blood flow. (16)

In one long term study 112 geriatric patients with chronic cerebral insufficiency were treated with Ginkgo biloba extract (GBE) at 120 mg/day for one year. Results showed that patients treated with GBE had significantly improved symptoms of cerebral insufficiency including improved symptoms of headache, vertigo, tinnitus, short term memory, vigilance and mood disturbance. (17) In another study of 166 geriatric patients with blood vessel disorders due to aging, GBE proved to be very effective. The effects of GBE became significant after 3 months of administration. Functional changes in electroencephalogram (EEG) were noted and patients experienced improved mental alertness. (18) In a study of 79 patients with arterial occlusive disease, GBE providd greater symptomatic relief than placebo. (19) In another study with 20 patients between the ages of 62 to 86 years with cerebral vascular insufficiency due to arteriosclerosis, dramatic improvement of cerebral blood flow was observed after only 2 weeks of GBE supplementation. (20)

Ginkgo biloba is safe and non-toxic and few adverse side effects have been reported. Stomach upset and headache have been reported in some individuals who consumed GBE in doses of up to 600 mg/day. Consumption of the fruit pulp of Ginkgo may cause allergic reactions including a topical red, itchy rash. (21)

RECOMMENDATIONS: Daily unless otherwise stated

Vitamin E...400 IU
Omega-3 Oil..5-10 gm
Ginkgo biloba (4:1)...120 mg

REFERENCES

(1) Acheson R et al: The Lancet pp. 1191-93, 1983
(2) Donahue RP et al: Alcohol and hemorrhagic stroke. The Honolulu Heart Program. JAMA. 255(17):2311-12, 1986
(3) Wilkins Mr et al: Stroke affecting young men after alcoholic binges. Brit. Med. J. 291:1342, 1985
(4) Littleton JM: Interactions between ethanol and dietary fat in determining human platelet function. Thromb. Haemost. 51(1):50-53, 1984
(5) Koganemaru S et al: The effect of vitamin E on platelet kinetics of stroke-prone spontaneously hypertensive rats. J. Nutr. Sci. & Vitaminology 29:1-10, 1982
(6) Black KL et al: Eicosapentaenoic acid: Effects on brain prostaglandins, cerebral blood flow and edema in ischemic gerbils. Stroke 15(1):65-69, 1984
(7) Foster S: Ginkgo. Botanical Series - 304. American Botanical Council. Austin, Texas, 1990
(8) Briancon-Scheid F et al: HPLC separation and quantitative determination of biflavones in leaves from ginkgo biloba. Planta Medica 49:204-7, 1983
(9) Borzeix MG et al: Recherches sure l'action antiagregant de l'extrait de ginkgo biloba.

Arch. Int. Pharmacodyn. 243:236, 1980

(10) Grosdemouge C et al: Effets de l'extrait de ginkgo biloba sure la rupture precoce de la barriere hemoencephalique le rat. Press Med. 15(31):1511, 1986

(11) Brunello N et al: Effects of an extract of ginkgo biloba on noradrenergic systems of rat cerebral cortex. Pharm. Res. Commun. 17:1063-72, 1985

(12) Pincemail J et al: Proprietes antiradicalaires de l`extrait de ginkgo biloba. Presse Med. 15(31):1475-79, 1986

13) Doly M et al: Effet de l'extrait de ginkgo biloba sur l'electrophysiologie de la retine isolee de rat diabetique. Presse Med. 15(31):1480-3, 1986

(14) Auguet M et al: Effects of an extract of ginkgo biloba on rabbit isolated aorta. Gen. Pharmac. 13:169, 1982

(15) Auguet M et al: Bases pharmacologiques de l'impact vasculaire de l'extrait de ginkgo biloba. Presse Med. 15(31):1524-8, 1986

(16) Massoni G et al: Effets microcirculatoieres de la ginkgo biloba chez les personnes agees. Giorn Geront. 20:444, 1972

(17) Voberg G: Ginkgo-biloba extract (GBE): A long term study of chronic cerebral vascular insufficiency in geriatric patients. Clin. Trials J. 22:149-57, 1985

(18) Taillandier J et al: Treatment of cerebral aging disorders with ginkgo biloba extract. Presse Med. 15(31):1583-7, 1986

(19) Bauer U: 6-month double-blind randomized clinical trial of ginkgo biloba extract versus placebo in two parallel groups suffering from peripheral arterial insufficiency. Arzneim-Forsch. 34:716-21, 1984

(20) Galley P et al: Tanakan et cerveau senile. Etude radiocirculographique. Bordeaux Med. 10:171, 1977

(21) Becker LE et al: Ginkgo-tree dermatits, stomatitis and proctitis. JAMA. 231:1162-3, 1975

CHAPTER 18

PROMOTING WEIGHT LOSS

Fifteen to 20% of North American adults are overweight and 5 to 8% of these adults are obese. Obesity is defined as excess of total body fat and is one of the most prevalent chronic disorders in the western hemisphere. Hypertension, heart disease, respiratory problems, non-insulin dependent diabetes (NIDDM), gall stones and cancer are among the major consequences of being overweight, especially those with severe obesity. It has long been recognized that obesity and weight control problems run in families. Both genetic and and environmental factors are contributory to overeating and weight gain. The causes and development of weight gain and obesity are multifactorial involving many factors including genetic, behavioral and psychosocial factors. Energy imbalances   created when energy intake exceeds energy expenditure is the fundamental mechanism leading to weight gain. In North America the typical diet is composed of 40 to 45% carbohydrates, 15 to 20% protein and 40% fat. A more ideal diet would be 60% carbohydrate, 15 to 20% protein and 20% fat. In addition, a sedentary lifestyle devoid of activity and exercise results in minimal caloric expenditure and contributes to energy imbalance.

Regular activity and physical exercise should be a major part of any weight control program. The management of mild to moderate weight problems should be diverse and should include dietary, nutritional, physical and psychosocial factors. Nutritional education and improved nutritional understanding contributes to weight control and results from effective and practical dietary counselling. Behavior modification has proven to be an effective part of a weight management program. The use of appetite suppressing drugs are only moderately effective in the treatment of obesity and are of little or no help in maintaining long term weight loss. Dietary, nutritional and botanical medicines can provide effective support for weight loss.

DIET

Caloric expenditure should exceed dietary caloric intake. A low calorie diet together with increased physical activity and exercise should be the foundation of any dietary program. A high fiber diet increases non-caloric bulk to cause appetite suppression and leads to less food intake. (1) Supplementation with Glucomannan, an unabsorbable complex carbohydrate from Konjak root, results in significant weight loss despite no changes in eating and exercise patterns. (2) Guar gum, another unabsorbable carbohydrate reduced hunger in obese subjects and influenced carbohydrate and fat metabolism in a beneficial manner contributing to weight loss. (3) An increased dietary consumption of raw foods leads to significant weight loss in obese hypertensive individuals. (4) The results of several studies suggest that sugar ingestion can lead to calorie over-consumption and obesity. (5) There is however, insufficient evidence to conclude that obese individuals consume a greater proportion of carbohydrates as compared to lean people.

NUTRIENTS

One controlled study of ascorbic acid (Vitamin C) in obesity showed that supplementation of vitamin C alone with no caloric restriction resulted in significant weight loss when compared to placebo. (6)

Coenzyme Q10 may be deficient in obese individuals and supplementation results in weight loss. (7)

Evening primrose oil (EPO) is believed to increase brown fat and Na/K ATPase activity and benefit people who fail to lose weight with appropriate diets (estimated to be 1 out 3 obese individuals). Supplementation with essential fatty acids results in significant weight loss. (8)

The amino acid L-Glutamine may decrease carbohydrate craving. L-Glutamine is able to cross the blood-brain barrier where it is able to be converted to Glutamic acid, a neurotransmitter in the brain. (9)

L-Tryptophan supplementation may reduce late night binging.

Tryptophan helps to increase serotonin levels which influence moods and inhibits appetite(10)

BOTANICAL MEDICINES

Ma Huang (Ephedra sinensis) is a native shrub of mainland China that has been used medicinally for over 5000 years in the treatment of respiratory infections, asthma and hayfever. Ephedra was introduced in western medicine in 1924. Ephedra contains 1.0 to 3.0% total alkaloid content as ephedrine, pseudoephedrine and norpseudoephedrine as its active ingredients. Ephedrine has important effects on intermediate metabolism. Ephedrine and related alkaloids have sympathomimetic activity that activates the sympathetic nervous system. Human fat cells contain alpha-2 receptors that when activated inhibit fat breakdown by decreasing intracellular cAMP. Human fat cells also contain beta-1 receptors that when activated increase fat breakdown. Ephedrine and related alkaloids activate beta-1 receptors and stimulate fat breakdown in fat cells. Ephedrine also enhances breakdown of sugar in the liver which leads to increased glucose release into circulation. Compared to adrenaline, another sympathomimetic, ephedrine has a longer duration of action, greater oral activity, more pronounced central effects and much lower potency. Ephedrine has shown to increase weight loss in experimental animal models. (11, 12, 13)

Green tea (Camellia sinensis) has been widely used in China for nearly 3000 years for its stimulant effects. The major difference between green tea and black tea is that green tea is made from leaves steamed and dried, while black tea leaves are withered, rolled, fermented and dried. Dried and cured leaves from this plant contain 3.0 to 5.0% methylxanthines primarily as caffeine. In addition, Camellia sinensis also contains a high concentration of tannins responsible for the astringent and stomach irritating effects of tea and coffee. In low and moderate doses the methylxanthines, especially caffeine, cause mild cortical arousal with increased alertness and delay of fatigue. In unusually sensitive individuals the caffeine contained in one cup of coffee, approximately 100 to 150 mg of caffeine per cup, is sufficient to cause nervousness and insomnia. Caffeine is a central nervous stimulant (CNS) and increases metabolic rate and activates beta-2 receptors which increases fat breakdown in fat cells. (11,14)

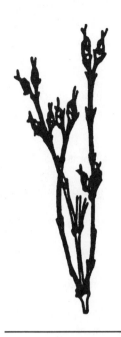
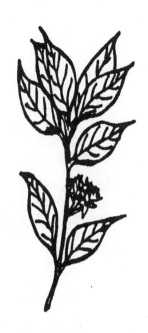

Ma Huang (Ephedra sinensis)   Kola (Cola nitida)

Kola (Cola nitida) is a tree native to parts of Africa whose wood is white, sometimes slightly pink when fresh and is valued for its used in woodwork and carpentry. The nuts of Cola nitida are used in West Africa to sustain people during long journeys or during long hours of work. In parts of the tropics where it grows, the fresh nut is chewed as a stimulant similar to betelnut. Africans believe that Cola nitida is an aphrodisiac in males and promotes conception in females. Cola nitida contains no less than 1.0% caffeine, usually about 3.5% and nearly 1.0% theobromine. The three most important methylxanthines are theophylline, theobromine and caffeine. Methylxanthines are potent central nervous system stimulants that increase basal metabolic rate and promote fat breakdown by activating beta-1 receptors on fat cells. (11, 14, 15)

RECOMMENDATIONS: Daily unless otherwise stated

Vitamin C...3000-5000 mg
Coenzyme Q10..100 mg
Evening Primrose Oil...2-5 gm

L-Glutamine..................................500-1000 mg
Ephedra sinensis (4:1)..........................400-800 mg
Camellia sinensis (4:1)..........................400-800 mg
Cola nitida (4:1)..................................400-800 mg

REFERENCES

(1) Cereal Foods World 29-11:635

(2) Walsh DE et al: Effect of glucomannan on obese patients: A clinical study. Int. J. Obes. 8(4):289-93, 1984

(3) Krotkiewski M: Effect of guar gum on body weight, hunger ratings and metabolism in obese subjects. Br. J. Nutr. 52(1):97-105, 1984

(4) Douglass J et al: Effects of a raw food diet on hypertension and obesity. South. Med. J. 78(7)84, 1985

(5) Vasselli JR: Carbohydrate injestion, hypoglycemia and obesity. Appetite 6:53-59, 1985

(6) Naylor GJ et al: A double blind placebo controlled trial of ascorbic acid in obesity. Nutr. Health, p. 425, 1985

(7) van Gaal L et al: Exploratory study of coenzyme Q10 in obesity. Biomed. & Clin Aspects of Coenzyme Q. Vol. 4. Amsterdam, Elsevier Science Publishers, pp. 369-73, 1984

(8) Lowndes RH et al: The effects of evening primrose oil (Efamol) on serum ipid levels of normal and obese subjects. Clinical Uses of Essential Fatty Acids. Montreal, Eden Press, pp. 37-52, 1982

(9) Williams RJ: Nutrition Against Disease, Pitman Publishing Co., New York, NY, 1971

(10) Goodwin F: Nat. Instit. of Mental Health - quoted in APA Psychiatric News, December 5, 1986

(11) Duke JA: Handbook of Medicinal Herbs: CRC press. Boca Raton, FL, 1985

(12) Gilman AG et al: The Pharmacologic Basis of Therapeutics. MacMillan Publishing, New York, NY, 1980

(13) Zarrindaat MR et al: Anorectic effects of ephedrine. Gen. Pharmacol. 18:559-61, 1987

(14)Leung AY: Encyclopedia of Common Natural Ingredients Used in Food, Drugs, and Cosmetics. John Wiley & Sons, 1980

(15) Tyler V. et al: Pharmacognosy, 8th edition. Lea & Febiger. Philadelpia, Pennsylvania, 1981

CHAPTER 19

QUITTING CIGARETTE SMOKING

Cigarette smoking is a common substance abuse problem in society and represents the greatest, single cause of chronic illness, disability and death in North America. Overall, the prevalence of smoking remains approximately 35% in men and 29% in women. One estimate suggests that each cigarette smoked results in a loss of five minutes of life, averaging five to eight years lost in smokers versus non-smokers. One in seven deaths in North America is directly related to cigarette smoking. Diseases related to smoking include, cardiovascular disease including heart attack and stroke, lung cancer, chronic obstructive pulmonary disease (COPD), asthma and development of peptic ulcers and alzheimer's disease. Smoking is associated with serious problems in the pregnant female, including a low birth-weight child, growth retardation and sudden infant death syndrome (SIDS).

Approximately 60 to 80% of smokers who attempt to quit achieve a minimal period of abstinence. However, the rate of relapse is high and approximately two-thirds of quitters resume smoking in three to six months and often within only a few days after quitting. Only 15 to 20% of quitters remain cigarette free for six months or more. Health benefits of smoking cessation are dramatic. The greatest immediate benefit of smoking cessation is reduction in the risk of developing cardiovascular disease. The financial benefits of smoking cessation are a further impetus to quit the habit. A person smoking one pack a day is probably spending close to $1000 per year on cigarettes alone. If this money was invested in an RRSP (Registered Retirement Saving Plan) from age 25 to the age of retirement, over 1.6 million dollars would have been accumulated. Smoking is the single most common cause of preventable disease. Quitting smoking is on the best improvements in health that a smoker can take. Dietary and nutritional support is available for helping individuals curb this addiction and quit this deadly habit.

PSYCHOLOGY

The most important factor in any stop smoking program is the desire to quit. The reason for smoking should be clearly identified and explored. Reasons include, a habit, psychologic addiction, a means of reducing tension, pleasurable relaxation, enjoyment of handling a cigarette or stimulation. Suggestions to modify behavior should be made and should include the following considerations:

- Switch to a filter cigarette or distasteful brand.
- Don't carry cigarettes, buy a limited number and put them out after a few inhalations.
- Smoke only in unpleasant circumstances.
- Try to quit one day at a time
- Substitute gardening, new recipes, exercise, movies, bike riding, walking, etc...as a substitute for smoking.
- Buy something to reward yourself for not smoking.
- Don't empty ashtrays, in order to create an unpleasant association with cigarette smoking.
- Avoid alcohol and other things or circumstances associated with cigarette smoking.
- Substitute toothpicks or other objects for cigarettes.
- Induce someone else to quit smoking at the same time.
- Start a diet with a self-improvement program simultaneously.

Continual encouragement and support should be provided during the initial course of abstinence.

NUTRIENTS

Vitamin A and Beta-carotene are required for development and maintenance of the integrity of connective tissue in the membranes of the throat and lungs. (1) Furthermore, Beta-carotene acts as an antioxidant and may protect the lungs and other tissues from the damaging toxins present in cigarette smoke. (2)

Decreased levels of Vitamin C is associated with cigarette smoking. (3) Vitamin C acts as an antioxidant and is involved in connective tissue integrity and the immune system.

Supplementation with Vitamin E and Selenium, both potent antioxidants, may be beneficial. (4)

BOTANICAL MEDICINES

Green oats (Avena sativa) has been traditionally used as a muscle relaxant and antidepressant. Green oats has been used successfully in India to cure opium addiction and has been reported to reduce the craving for tobacco. (5) Although the active ingredients in Avena have not been identified, Avena is known to contain steroidal saponins, flavonoids and alkaloids. (6) In one double blind study an alcoholic extract of Avena sativa was used to successfully treat 26 cigarette smokers. Each patient kept a daily record of the number of cigarettes smoked. After 6 months, the results of the Avena treated group versus placebo were compared. The Avena treated group had a significant decrease in the number of cigarettes smoked. 25% of those treated with Avena quit smoking altogether. And although the patients made no conscious effort to quit smoking, they reported various degrees of loss of craving for cigarettes. Moreover, the reduction in smoking continued even two months after termination of the Avena program. (7) An effort to elucidate the pharmacologic actions of Avena sativa reported that constituents in Avena antagonized morphine effects in mice. Avena was further found to antagonize the blood vessel constrictive response in blood pressure regulation by nicotine. (8)

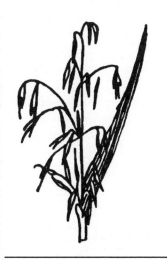
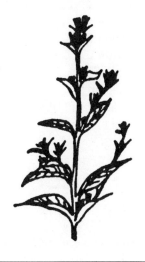

Green Oats (Avena sativa)   Lobelia (Lobelia inflata)

Indian tobacco (Lobelia inflata) is a hairy annual or biennial herb, growing up to 1 meter high and is native to parts of North America. Lobelia contains 0.48% piperidine alkaloids composed mainly of lobeline. (9) Lobeline has been reported to have many of the pharmacological activities of nicotine, although it is one-third as potent as nicotine. (10) Like nicotine it first stimulates the central nervous system (CNS) followed by severe CNS depression. Lobelia has been traditionally used as antispasmodic, antiasthmatic, diaphoretic, expectorant, emetic and sedative. The American Indians used lobelia as a tobacco substitute. Lobelia containing the alkaloid lobeline is an effective antagonist to nicotine from tobacco, though much less potent. Lobelia may be used as a substitute for cigarette smoking. In the United States the FDA has allowed the sale of pills containing lobeline to be used as a smoking deterrent ("Washington Post", January 11, 1982). Lobeline can be very toxic in large doses. The list of toxicity include depression, nausea, sweats, stupor, depression, progressive vomiting, weakness, prostration, convulsions and coma. Excessive ingestion of lobeline can cause respiratory paralysis and can be fatal. (11) Lobelia containing lobeline can be used effectively as a smoking deterrent, but discretion should be exercised in regards to the potentially toxic side effects of this plant

RECOMMENDATIONS: Daily unless otherwise stated

Vitamin A..50,000-100,000 IU
Beta-carotene...200 mg
Vitamin C..1000-3000 mg
Vitamin E..400 IU
Zinc...25-50 mg
Selenium...400 mcg
Avena sativa (10:1)...400-800 mg
Lobelia inflata (4:1)...400-800 mg

REFERENCES

(1) Guyton AC: Textbook of Medical Physiology. WB Saunders Company, Philadelphia, Penn. 1986
(2) Burton G et al: Beta-carotene: An unusual type of antioxidant. Science 224:569-73, 1984

(3) Pelletier O: Smoking and vitamin C levels in humans. AM. J. Clin. Nutr. 21:1259-67, 1968

(4) Combs GF: Assessment of vitamin E status in animals and man. Proc. Nutr. Soc. 40:187-94, 1981

(5) Anand CL: Treatment of Opium Addiction. Brit. Med. J. 3:641, 1971

(6) Tschesche R et al: Chem. Ber. 102:2072, 1969

(7) Anand CL: Effect of Avena sativa on cigarette smoking. Nature Vol. 233:496, Ocotber 15, 1971

(8) Connor J et al: The pharmacology of Avena sativa. J. Pharm. Pharmac. 27:92-98, 1975

(9) Leung A: Encyclopedia of Common Natural Ingredients Used in Food, Drugs, and Cosmetics. John Wiley & Sons, New York, NY, 1980

(10) Gilman A et al: Thr Pharmacological Basis of Therapeutics. MacMillan Publ. New York, NY, 1980

(11) Duke JA: Hanbook of Medicinal Herbs, CRC Press, Boca Raton, FL. 1985

CHAPTER 19

REDUCING PROSTATE ENLARGEMENT

Prostate enlargement, otherwise known as benign prostatic hyperplasia (BPH) is estimated to affect 50% of men over the age of 50 and increases with increasing age. Symptoms of BPH include increased frequency of urination, urination at night, incomplete bladder emptying, inability to void, overflow incontinence and terminal dribbling. BPH is caused by an abnormal enlargement of the prostate gland which irritates the bladder and the urethra. The prostate gland contributes to seminal fluid a secretion containing acid phosphatase, citric acid and proteolytic enzymes which account for the liquefaction of the semen. The rate of secretion normally increases during sexual stimulation. When the prostate gland abnormally enlarges it impinges on the bladder and urethra and subsequently, leads to many of the symptoms associated with BPH. The exact cause of BPH is unknown, but hormonal imbalances are known to play an important role in its development. There is no effective medical treatment and prostate surgery remains the mainstay of conventional therapy. There are safe and effective natural alternatives that should be explored before surgery is done.

NUTRIENTS

Zinc supplementation may be beneficial. In one experimental study zinc supplementation reduced the size of the prostate and significantly improved symptoms in a majority of patients. (1) Fourteen of 19 patients who received 150 mg of zinc as zinc sulphate for 2 months had a significant reduction in prostate size. (2)

The amino acids glutamic acid, alanine and glycine taken as L-form amino acids may also be beneficial. One study of 45 patients who were supplemented with glutamic acid, alanine and glycine, had significant improvement of the symptoms associated with BPH. (3)

Essential fatty acid supplementation may also be beneficial. When the hormone testosterone enters prostate cells it is converted to dihydrotestosterone which enters the cell nucleus and stimulates protein synthesis and cell growth. Testosterone also stimulates prostaglandin synthesis. It has been postulated that released prostaglandins bind testosterone receptors which inhibit further testosterone binding and uptake into prostate cells. Aging causes decreased efficiency of prostaglandin synthesis and hence, decreased receptor binding. Subsequently, more testosterone is able to bind membrane receptors, enter the cell and stimulate protein synthesis and cell growth. (4) Essential oils are precursors to prostaglandins and supplementation may stimulate prostaglandin synthesis and counteract the deficiency caused by aging. (5)

Cadmium exposure and toxicity may result in BPH, while Selenium may protect against Cadmium induced prostate enlargement. (6,7)

BOTANICAL MEDICINES

Stinging nettle (Urtica dioica) has been used medicinally for it's characteristic sting in Europe, Asia and North America. The steroidal component of stinging nettle inhibits prostatic enlargement. Stinging nettle extract inhibits androgenic hormone binding to the surface of prostate cells. It also inhibits sodium-potassium enzyme activity which subsequently suppresses prostate cell metabolism and growth. It may also affect prostaglandin production which alters prostatic growth and enlargement. (8,9,10)

The bark of the African tree Pygeum africanum has been used treat benign prostatic hyperplasia in both Europe and Africa. Sterols in the bark are believed to inhibit the enzyme 5-alpha reductase which is responsible for converting testosterone to dihydrotestosterone. In one clinical study of 263 patients with prostate enlargement those patients that use the extract of Pygeum showed significant improvement in urinary symptoms. In another clinical study of 134 patients with prostate enlargement there was significant improvement in the Pygeum treated patients in terms of urinary flow, residual urine and night time frequency. (11,12)

Saw palmetto (Serenoa repens) is a small dwarf tree native to the West Indies and the south-east coast of North America. The Indians used the berries of this plant for food and medicinally to treat a variety of respiratory and genito-urinary illness. It has been used to treat colds, bronchitis, asthma, irritated mucousal membranes, chronic and subacute cystitis and prostate complaints in men. Saw palmetto has been reputed to be an aphrodisiac. While this last claim is unsubstantiated, Saw palmetto berry extracts have been used successfully to treat benign prostate hyperplasia. (13)

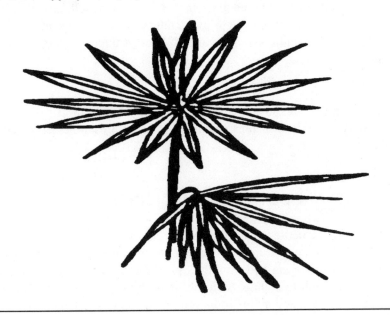

Saw palmetto (Serenoa repens)

Saw palmetto berries contain about 1.5% of an oil composed of free fatty acids and ethyl esters of these acids. Other constituents of the berries include tannins, resins, lipase and a variety of sugars. (13) A purifeid Saw palmetto extract containing 85 to 95% fatty acid content has been used to treat BPH.

The concentrated oil extract from Saw palmetto berries has been shown to inhibit the enzyme 5-Alpha-reductase which is responsible for the converion of testosterone to dihydrotestosterone. The concentrated oil extract called a liposterolic extract, also inhibits dihydrotestosterone binding to nuclear receptors. The net outcome is that the liposterolic extract from Saw palmetto berries prevents protein synthesis and cell growth, thereby preventing prostate enlargement. (14,15)

   In a study of 110 outpatients with prostate enlargement, 55 were treated with a liposterolic extract from Saw palmetto berries versus the other 55 who received a placebo for 30 days. The group treated with the liposterolic extract showed significant improvement in the symptoms associated with prostate enlargement. The liposterolic extract was well tolerated and no side effects were reported. Researchers concluded that the liposterolic extract from Saw palmetto berries was effective in treating prostate enlargement. (16)

   The liposterolic extract from Saw palmetto berries is well tolerated and no side effects have been reported. (16)

RECOMMENDATIONS: Daily unless otherwise stated

Zinc..50-100 mg
Selenium..400 mcg
L-glutamic acid, L-alanine, L-glycine.............................2-4 gm
Essential oils..5-10 gm
Urtica dioica extract..500-1000 mg
Pygeum africanum (4:1)......................................100-200 mg
Serenoa repens (80-95% liposterolic extract)..................320 mg

REFERENCES

(1) Fahim M et al: Zinc treatment for the reduction of hyperplasia of the prostate. Fed. Proc. 35:361, 1976
(2) Bush IM et al: Zinc and the prostate. AMA annual meeting. Chicago, 1974
(3) Dumrau F: Benign prostatic hyperplasia: Amino acid therapy for symptomatic relief. Am. J. Ger. 10:426-30, 1962
(4) Klein La et al: Prostaglandins and the prostate. Prostate 4(3): 247-51, 1983
(5) Hart JP et al: Vitamin F in the treatment of prostatic hyperplasia. Report No. 1, Lee Foundation for Nutritional Research, Milwaukee, WI, 1941
(6) Habib FK et al: Metal-androgen interrelationships in carcinoma and hyperplasia of the human prostate. J. Endocrinol. 71(1):133-41, 1976
(7) Webber MM: Selenium prevents the growth stimulatory effects of cadmium on human prostate epithelium. Biochem. Biophy. Res. Commun. 127(3):871-77, 1985
(8) Hirano T et al: Effects of stinging nettle root extracts and their steroidal components on Na-K ATPase of the nbenign prostatic hyperplasia. Planta Medica, 60(1):30-3, 1994

February
(9) Vahlensieck W Jr et al: Drug therapy of benign prostatic hyperplasia. Fortschr Med, 113(31):407-11 1996 Nov 10
(10) Hryb DJ et al: The effect of extracts of the roots of the stinging nettle (Urtica dioica) on the interaction of SHBG with its receptor on human prostatic membranes. Planta Med, 61(1):31-2, 1995 Feb
(11) Krzeski T et al: Combine extracts of Urtica dioica and Pygeum africanum in the treatment of enign prostatic hyperplasia, Clin Ther, 15(6):1011-20, 1993 Nov-Dec
(12) Barlet A et al: Efficacy of Pygeum africanum extract in the medical therpy of urination disorders due to benign prostatic hyperplasia: evaluation of objective and subjective parameters. A placebo-controlled double-blind multicenter study. Wien Klin Wochenschr, 102(22):667-73 1990 Nov 23m
(13) Duke JA: Handbook of Medicinal Herbs. CRC press, Boca Raton, Fl. 1985
(14) Carilla E et al: Binding of Permixon, a new treatment for prostatic benign hyperplasia, to the cytosolic androgen receptor in the rat prostate. J. Steroid Biochem. 20:521-3, 1984
(15) Sultan C et al: Inhibition of androgen metabolism and binding by a liposterolic extract of "Serneoa repens B" in human foreskin fibroblasts. J. Steroid Biochem. 20:519-9, 1984
(16) Champlault G et al: A double-blind trial of an extract of the plant Serenoa repens in benign prostatic hyperplasia. Br. J. Clin. Pharmacol. 18:461-2, 1984

CHAPTER 21

RELAXING AN IRRITABLE BOWEL

Irritable bowel syndrome (IBS) is the most common cause of chronic diarrhea and lower abdominal discomfort. IBS is estimated to affect between 14 to 20% of the North American population with varying degrees of severity. Irritable bowel syndrome is the most common of all gastrointestinal disorders, accounting for 50 to 70% of all patients with digestive complaints. Symptoms of irritable bowel syndrome include nausea, abdominal bloating, abdominal pain, flatulence, diarrhea, constipation, anxiety and depression, all of which may be present from time to time. Onset of IBS commonly occurs in those individuals between the ages of 20 and 35. The cause of irritable bowel syndrome is unknown and treatment is only symptomatic. Safe and natural alternatives exist for the treatment of irritable bowel syndrome.

DIET

The addition of 10 to 30 grams of dietary fiber to the diet significantly improved abdominal discomfort, pain and bowel habit. (1) A diet composed of 30 grams of fruit and vegetable fiber and 10 grams of cereal fiber were compared. Both diets resulted in a significant improvement of the symptoms associated with IBS. (2) A diet high in refined carbohydrates has been implicated in the cause of IBS and certain other diseases of the colon. Spasm of the smooth muscle of the colon is the common pathogenic mechanism, while the strength of the spasm producing the increased pressure in the intestinal lumen and the wall of the colon and the length of time for which the colon has been affected are believed to affect the onset and severity of the disease. A diet high in refined carbohydrates intensifies the muscle spasm of the colon. Sugar should be avoided in the diet for those individuals suffering from IBS. (3)

Food sensitivities have also been implicated as possible triggering mechanisms. Patients placed on a diet eliminating frequently incriminated foods for two weeks benefited and were able to identify offending foods upon their re-introduction into the diet. (4) Wheat, milk, soy, beef, pork, food additives and colorings, corn, coffee, and citrus have been implicated as possible offending foods. (5)

NUTRIENTS

Supplementation with 40 to 60 mg of Folic acid per day has demonstrated to be beneficial for the treatment of chronic diarrhea. (6) In addition, hydrochloric acid supplementation has demonstrated to be effective in certain cases of chronic diarrhea. (7) Lactobacillus acidophilus supplementation may also be beneficial in certain cases of diarrhea. (8)

BOTANICAL MEDICINES

Peppermint (Mentha piperita), native to Europe and North America, is an aromatic perennial member of the mint family that grows up to one meter in height. Peppermint has been used traditionally for centuries to treat a variety of gastrointestinal disorders. (9)

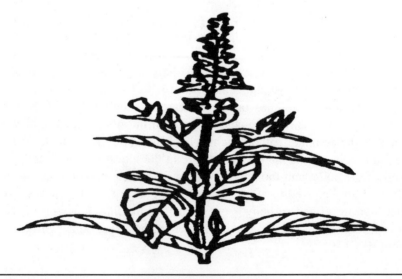

Peppermint (Mentha piperita)

Peppermint leaves contain up to 2.0% volatile oil containing menthol, menthone and jasmone, that has been identified as the active ingredient in this plant. (10)

Peppermint oil directly inhibits gastrointestinal smooth muscle contractions and is helpful in preventing intestinal spasming. Peppermint oil has been used to treat stomach cramping, relieve heartburn and relax the lower esophageal sphincter. Peppermint oil has been used widely as a counter-irritant on the skin and as an antipruritic, to relieve itching. In addition, peppermint oil has demonstrated antimicrobial activity against bacteria, viruses and fungi. (11)

Peppermint oil has demonstrated remarkable effectiveness in alleviating many of the symptoms associated with irritable bowel syndrome. Patients who ingested 3 to 6 capsules per day, at 0.2 ml of peppermint oil per capsule, were relieved of their symptoms. (12) In one British hospital enteric-coated peppermint oil capsules are being used to reduce colon spasm during intestinal endoscopy. Colon spasm was relieved remarkably fast in 20 patients who underwent this diagnostic procedure. (13) Antispasmodic drugs are usually given intravenously in this procedure which is uncomfortable to the patient while enteric-coated peppermint oil may be taken orally without any problems. Peppermint oil capsules must be enteric-coated to prevent premature oil release and rapid absorption in the upper digestive tract. Enteric-coating prevents digestion of the capsules and allows them to be released in the small and large intestine. Enteric-coated peppermint oil is remarkably effective in treating the symptoms of irritable bowel syndrome. (14)

Peppermint oil is safe and generally non-toxic. Peppermint oil may be irritating to the skin, eyes and other mucous membranes. Internally, peppermint oil can be irritating to the intestinal tract in high doses and can exert a depressant effect on the heart. (10)

RECOMMENDATIONS: Daily unless otherwise stated

Folic acid..40-60 mg
HCl supplements...3-6 caps
Lactobacillus acidophilus..1-2 tsp
Mentha piperita (enteric-coated capsules)...............0.6-1.2 ml

REFERENCES

(1) Cann P et al: What is the benefit of coarse wheat bran in patients with irritable bowel syndrome? Gut 25:168-73, 1984

(2) Fielding J et al: Different dietary fibre formulations and the irritable bowel syndrome. Irish J. Med. Sci. 153:178-80, 1984

(3) Grimes DS: Refined carbohydrate, smooth-muscle spasm and diseases of the colon. Lancet 1:395-97, 1976

(4) Alun Jones V et al: Food intolerance in irritable bowel syndrome. Clin. Ecology 3(1):35-8, 1985

(5) Alun Jones V et al: Food intolerance: A major factor in the pathogenesis of irritable bowel syndrom. Lancet 2:1115-7, 1982

(6) Carruthers LB: Chronic diarrhea treated with folic acid. Lancet 1:849, 1946

(7) Bulletin Gen. de Therapeutique, Paris - abstracted in JAMA 39:55, 1902

(8) Niv M et al: Yogurt in the treatment of infantile diarrhea. Clin Ped. 2:407-11, 1963

(9) Foster S: Peppermint Mentha x piperita. American Botanical Council, Austin, Texas, 1990

(10) Leung AY: Encyclopedia of Common Natural Ingredients Used in Food, Drugs, and Cosmetics, John Wiley & Sons, New York, NY, 1980

(11) Weiss RF: Herbal Medicine: Beaconsfield Publishers Ltd. Beaconsfield, England, 1985

(12) Somerville KW et al: Delayed release peppermint oil capsules (Colpermin) for the spastic colon syndrome: A pharmacokinetic study. Br. J. Clin. Pharmac. 18:638-40, 1984

(13) Leicester R et al: Peppermint oil to reduce colonic spasm during endoscopy. Lancet ii:989, 1980

(14) Rees W et al: Treating irritable bowel syndrome with peppermint oil. Br. Med. J. ii:835-6, 1979

CHAPTER 22

RELIEVING MENOPAUSAL SYMPTOMS

Menopause refers to the condition when the ovaries stop functioning and both menstruation and childbearing cease. Menopause is often called "change of life" or "climacteric" and occurs to all women throughout the world. Menopause is a natural physiologic process that results from normal aging of the ovaries. When the ovaries stop functioning many of the symptoms of menopause occur. The most common symptoms associated with menopause is hot flashes. 60 to 75% of women going through menopause experience hot flushes to the face, neck and upper body. They may also experience excessive perspiration, especially at night. Hot flushes typically last from 30 to 60 seconds in duration, can occur at virtually any time and can reoccur over 50 times per day. Decreased menstrual flow, decreased bleeding during the period and periods spaced further apart are usually the first signs of menopause. Other symptoms include fatigue, insomnia, dizziness, tingling in extremities, rapid heart beat, heart palpitations, difficult and painful sexual intercourse, inability to hold urine, bladder infections, vaginitis, dry vagina, nausea, bloating, gas, flatulence, constipation, muscle and joint pain. It is interesting to note that 15% of women pass through menopause without experiencing any symptoms at all. Decreased size of the ovaries, fallopian tubes, uterus and vagina occurs. Osteoporosis or decreased bone mass can occur as a consequence of menopause. Menopause generally last from one to five years in duration, although hot flushes for more than ten years have been reported

Conventional medical treatment of menopause consists of the use of antidepressants, muscle relaxants and hormone therapy. T h e main concerns of about synthetic hormone therapy are the negative side effects of these hormones. The most serious side effect of estrogen therapy is the increased risk factor of breast and uterine cancer. Any women that is considering hormone therapy should be screened and monitored about the possible risk of these cancers. If there is a strong possibility or family history for these cancers that conventional hormone therapy should be discouraged. Other adverse effects of estrogen therapy include nausea, vomiting, headaches, high blood pressure, jaundice gallstones, fluid retention, edema, swelling, gas, bloating, blood sugar abnormalities, blood clots, thrombophlebitis, breast pain, fibrocystic breast disease, fibroids, endometriosis and mood changes. (4,5,6) While synthetic progesterone is not currently considered as cancer promoting, it is not without adverse side effects. Adverse side effects of synthetic progesterone include salt and water retention, swelling, edema, high blood pressure, abdominal gas and bloating, weight gain, nausea, vomiting, skin rashes, insomnia, mood changes, memory problems, irritability, depression, abnormal vaginal bleeding, jaundice, liver disease, blood clots, thrombophlebitis, and clots in the lungs. (4,5,6)

LIFESTYLE

Menopause can be a particularly stressful time of life. If stress is an obvious factor in your life then a stress evaluation is warranted. Stressors should be identified and eliminated if possible. Concerns, fears and questions regarding menopause should be addressed. Any misconceptions about menopause should be corrected. Menopause is a normal, natural consequence of aging that occurs to all women throughout the world. Some women experience unpleasant side effects that can be effectively managed using natural therapies. Menopause does not only happen to old, neurotic women. Menopause does not make a women less sexy or less beautiful. You can still enjoy a fulfilling sex life during and after menopause. And additionally, many women fell that they are freed of the burden and responsibilities of pregnancy and childbirth. (4) Moderate aerobic exercise helps to reduce symptoms of menopause. Exercise should be incorporated into daily routine. It is a great way to reduce stress, improve moods, improve physical fitness and reduce hot flushes. A routine of walking, swimming, bicycling or other form of aerobic exercise should be done for 20 to 30 minutes per day. (4,11) Synthetic clothe fibers can aggravate symptoms of menopause, particularly hot flushes. Natural fibers, including cotton, should be used for clothing choices as often as possible.

DIET

A diet high in caffeine containing foods and beverages is known to increase the symptoms of menopause, including hot flushes. Coffee should be eliminated altogether or only 1-2 cups consumed per day. Other caffeine containing foods and beverages should be consumed only in moderation. Avoid white sugar and refined carbohydrates. Decrease consumption of fats including red meat, dairy and processed foods. Increase consumption of whole, unprocessed foods, fresh fruits and vegetables. Increased consumption of foods high in vitamin E including whole grains and cereals, wheat germ, nuts and seeds. Increase consumption of fresh, unsweetened vegetable and fruits juices.

Specifically increase consumption of soy beans and soy derivatives including tofu. Soybeans are rich in natural chemicals called flavones that dramatically improve symptoms of menopause including hot flushes. Flavones are believed to interact like estrogen in the brain of menopausal females by inhibiting the release of FSH and LH. Researcher believe that a diet high in soybeans by Asian women directly contributes to their decreased incidence of menopause and breast cancer. Soybeans and tofu are also an excellent source of calcium and other nutrients. Also increase consumption of yams. Yams are a rich source of steroidal chemicals that resemble estrogen and progesterone. The can interact with the hormonal system and can inhibit the release of FSH and LH. (4,12,13)

VITAMIN AND MINERALS

Vitamin A or Beta carotene helps to maintain the lining of the vagina and uterus. It also acts as a potent antioxidant and improves immune function.

Vitamin B-complex help to maintain a healthy nervous system. B-complex vitamins are widely referred to as "the stress vitamins." During periods of stress we require a slightly higher intake of B vitamins. During menopause stress level can increase dramatically and supplementation with B-complex vitamins may be beneficial. Vitamin B5 or Pantothenic acid helps to support the nervous system and the functioning of the adrenal glands. Vitamin B6 or pyridoxine is used by the liver in many enzymatic reactions. It is used to help breakdown estrogen and other female hormones. It is also used to help break down toxins.

Vitamin C or ascorbic acid may be deficient. Supplementation may help to decrease hot flashes and improve other symptoms of menopause.

Vitamin E supplementation may help to decrease hot flushes and improve other symptoms of menopause. Intravaginal insertion of a vitamin E capsule can help to improve vaginal dryness and irritation. (14,15)

Boron is a relatively unknown trace mineral that is required by the body in small amounts. Boron is required by the liver to activate steroid hormone, including estrogen. It may also be necessary to activate vitamin D to its active form. No RDA for boron has been established. Current research indicates that the daily requirement for this mineral is 1 to 3 milligrams per day. Boron appears to be relatively non-toxic and few adverse side effects have been reported. (16)

Calcium is necessary for the development and maintenance of healthy bones. Calcium supplementation may help to improve certain symptoms of menopause including fatigue, muscle spasms and abdominal cramps. Calcium supplementation is useful in preventing the development of osteoporosis. (17)

Magnesium supplementation may help to improve certain symptoms of menopause including fatigue, muscle cramps, abdominal cramps and depression. (17)

FOOD SUPPLEMENTS

Bee pollen consist of plant pollens collected by worker bees and is combined with plant nectar and bee saliva. The pollen is packed into small pellets and is used as a food source for male drones. Bee pollen consists of protein, amino acids, sugars and a small amount of vitamins, minerals and enzymes. A partially fermented bee pollen produce under the trade name "Melbrosia " has been used in Europe for over 30 years to treat menopause. Few clinical studies have been performed to document the use of this product, but many individuals attest to its effectiveness. It should be noted that bee pollen products contain small amounts of plant pollens and should be consumed with caution in allergy sensitive individuals.

Evening primrose oil (Oenothera biennis) is a beautiful flowering plant of the Nightshade family and is native to many parts of North America. The seeds of this plant contain from 2 to 5% oils. Up to 76% of the oils is in the form of omega-6 oils. Omega-6 oils are an essential oil that must be obtained in a small amount on a daily basis for good health. Omega-6 oils have many important biological functions in the human body. One important function is that omega-6 oils are used to make prostaglandins. Prostaglandins are very powerful though short lived hormones that have strong effects throughout the body. Certain prostaglandins made from the omega-6 oil found in evening primrose seeds can reduce the symptoms of premenstrual stress and menopause. In the case of menopause these prostaglandins help to reduce the severity of hot flashes by reducing the production of FSH and LH hormones. (4)

Octacosanol is the name given to an oil extract that has been isolated from certain grains including rice germ and wheat germ. The oil extract exerts biological activity on the female reproductive system. Octacosanol supplementation can help to reduce the severity of symptoms associated with menopause. While no direct hormone activity of this oil extract has been implicated, octacosanol does affect endogenous reproductive hormones. Octacosanol is relatively safe and non-toxic. (13)

BOTANICAL MEDICINES

Scientific research is beginning to validate the use of certain medicinal plants in the treatment of various female disorders including menopause. Specific medicinal plants contain small amounts of steroid chemicals that resemble estrogen and progesterone. Those plant steroids resembling female hormones are called phytoestrogens. Phytoestrogens can exert a weak hormone effect on the body without actually altering the body's own estrogen and progesterone. Phytoestrogens are 1/400 as active as normal endogenous hormones produced in the ovaries. Phytoestrogens are believed to interact with the body's normal hormone feedback system. Phytoestrogens compete for binding sites on certain hormone sensitive cells. When natural estrogen levels are low in the body, phytoestrogens can bind to cell receptors and exert some hormonal activity. When estrogen levels are high, phytoestrogens compete with estrogen in the body for receptor binding sites.

Phytoestrogens can displace endogenous estrogen and limit it's biological actions. Certain plants contain phytoestrogens that interact with mostly estrogen receptors of the human. Other plants contain steroid precursors that interact with mostly progesterone receptors of the human body. Medicinal plants that are considered primarily estrogen sensitive are alfalfa, black cohosh, blue cohosh, dong quai, fennel, licorice and unicorn root. Medicinal plants that are considered to be primarily progesterone sensitive are chasteberry and wild yams. Phytoestrogen are generally considered safe and are not cancer promoting. The exact dose and prescription of a plant for treatment of menopause should be dependent on the active ingredients of the plant, the desired medicinal effect and patient sensitivity. (18,19)

Alfalfa (Medicago sativa) is a common leguminous plant resembling clover that is cultivated throughout the world as animal forage. Alfalfa contains 2.0 to 3.0% steroidal saponins, flavonoids, coumarin derivatives and alkaloids. Coumarin derivatives and the flavone tricin produce estrogen effects. Tricin relaxes smooth muscles of the uterus and is an antioxidant. Steroidal saponins produce a mild estrogenic effect, which explains this plants historical use for treating gynecological disorders. (20,21)

Black cohosh (Cimicifuga racemosa) is a perennial plant native to Europe and North America and has been used by american indians to treat a variety of female disorders. The root of this plant contains 15 to 20% of an oily resin called cimicifugin and steroid resembling chemicals called triterpene glycosides. One glycoside isolated from this plant called acteine has displayed mild estrogenic activity. A standardized extract containing a specified dose of acteine is one of the most widely prescribed medicinal plants in Germany and France. In clinical studies Black cohosh helps to reduce all symptoms of menopause as well as, if not better, than conventionally prescribed estrogen. This plant may contain a chemical similar to nicotine that can in large doses increase blood pressure and cause nausea, vomiting and dizziness. (22,23)

Blue cohosh (Caulophyllum racemosa) is a perennial herb with a thick crooked root, grows up to 1 metre in height and is native to eastern North America and parts of Europe. Blue cohosh contains steroid chemicals called triterpene glycosides and alkaloids. The glycosides exhibit mild estrogenic activity and can help to improve symptoms of menopause. The glycosides also have been found to prevent conception and cause uterine muscle contraction. The use of this plant during pregnancy is discouraged. Alkaloids in blue cohosh may be similar to nicotine and can increase blood pressure and can cause nausea, vomiting and dizziness. (22,23)

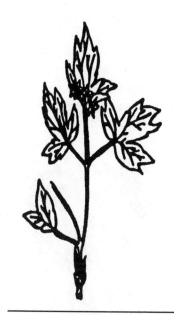

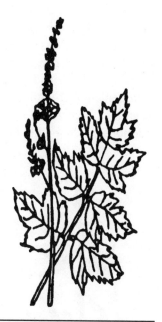

Blue Cohosh	Black Cohosh
(Caulophyllum thalictroides)	(Cimicifuga racemosa)

Chasteberry (Vitex agnus-castus) is a plant native to Mediterranean and central Asia. It was used in folk medicine to help suppress libido and prevent pregnancy. The fruits of this plant contains volatile oils that impart a distinct peppermint-like aroma. The volatile oil fractions interact with progesterone receptors in the body. It causes an increase in LH production and a decrease in FSH production. Most studies have used a whole plant extract in the form of a tincture with a dose of 40 drops once or twice per day. (25,26)

Dong quai (Angelica sinensis) is a stout perennial herb growing up to 2 metres in height and is native to mainland China and other parts of Asia. It has been used for thousands of years throughout the orient to treat a variety of female disorders including premenstrual syndrome, dysmenorrhea and menopause. It is commonly used as a female tonic and is second in popularity only to ginseng. The root and rhizome of this plant contain 0.3 to 1.0% volatile oils and 0.2% coumarin derivatives. The volatile oils account for the distinct odour of this plant and account for some of it's medicinal effects. Some of these medicinal effects include analgesic, anti-inflammatory, uterine smooth muscle relaxing, expectorant and immune stimulating effects. The coumarin derivative are believed to be responsible for the female effects of this plant. The coumarin derivatives appear to mimic the effects of estrogen on key centers in the brains of females. These coumarin derivatives are believed to bind to estrogen receptor sites in the hypothalamus and pituitary gland of the brain. By binding these receptor sites they exert a mild estrogenic effect without actually increasing endogenous estrogen. This negative feedback loop decreases the production of FSH and LH hormone production in the hypothalamus and pituitary gland. (22,27)

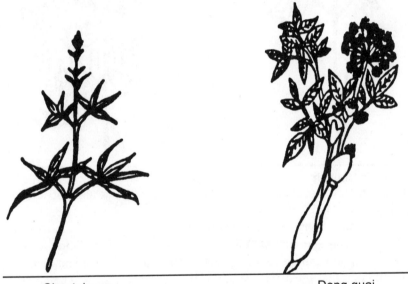

Chasteberry
(Vitex agnus castus)

Dong quai
(Angelica sinensis)

Fennel (Foeniculum vulgare) is an aromatic herb native to southern Europe, certain parts of Asia and is cultivated throughout North America. The "foeniculum" is derived from the latin word meaning fragrant. Fennel seeds contain 3 to 20% of a mixture of aromatic, volatile oils which account for its characteristic odour. Fennel has been used to increase milk production in lactating females, promote menstruation, facilitate easy childbirth, decrease menopausal symptoms and increase libido. The volatile oil fractions is believed to exert mild estrogenic effects in the body. Ingestion of a large amount of the oil can cause nausea, vomiting and skin rash. (22,24)

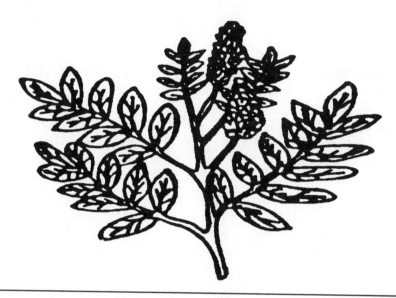

Licorice (Glycycrrhiza glabra)

Licorice (Glycyrrhiza glabra) is a perennial plant that grows 1 to 2 metres in height and is native to Asia, Europe and parts of the Middle East. Licorice root is widely used as a flavouring for candies and other confectionaries. The root contains 1 to 27% steroid chemicals called triterpene glycosides. The most common glycoside is called glycyrrhizin. Glycyrrhizin is at least 50 times more sweet than common table sugar. Glycyrrhizin produces a mild estrogen effect on the body of females. Licorice extracts are an excellent remedy for stomach and digestive problems. Large doses of licorice can cause electrolyte imbalance, swelling, edema, high blood pressure and diarrhea. These unpleasant side effects are eliminate with discontinued or decreased use of licorice. (26,27)

Mexican Yam (dioscorea mexicana) and other related yam species are a very rich source of natural steroid chemicals. Mexican yam is grown commercially for its steroid content and is used to make cortisone and oral contraceptives. Mexican yam contains up to 7% steroid chemicals; the most common of which is diosgenin. Diosgenin is similar in structure and function to progesterone. Although the human body does not possess the enzymes necessary to make progesterone from diosgenin, it does however exert biological activity. Wild yam preparations have been effectively used to control symptoms of menopause in both oral and topical forms. Yam preparations are relatively non-toxic and few side effects have been reported. (20,22)

RECOMMENDATIONS: Daily unless otherwise stated

Vitamin A...5,000-10,000 IU
Beta-carotene...10,000-25,000 IU
Vitamin B-complex..50 mg
Vitamin B5 (Pantothenic acid)...100-200 mg
Vitamin B6...10-25 mg
Vitamin C...250-500 mg
Vitamin E...400 IU
Calcium...800-1500 mg
Magnesium...400-750 mg
Alfalfa (4:1)..500-1000 mg
Black cohosh (4:1)..200-400 mg
Blue cohosh (4:1)..200-400 mg
Chasteberry (6:1)..200-400 mg
Dong quai (4:1)..500-1000 mg
Fennel (4:1)..75-150 mg
Licorice (4:1)...500-1000 mg
Mexican Yam (4:1)...500-1000 mg

REFERENCES

(1) Guyton AC: Textbook of Medical Physiology, W.B. Saunders, Philadelphia, Pennsylvania, pp. 968-92, 1986
(2) Jubiz, William: Endocrinology; Logical Approach for Clinicians, 2nd edition, McGraw-Hill Book Co., New York, NY, 1985
(3) Gaby, Alan R: Preventing and Reversing Osteoporosis, Prima Publishing, Rocklin Ca., 1994
(4) Kamen, Betty: Hormone Replacement Therapy: Yes or No? Nutrition Encounters Inc., Novato, CA., 1993
(5) Gambrell RD Jr: Complications of estrogen therapy. In Hormone Replacement Therapy, edited by D.P. Swartz, Chapter 9, Williams and Wilkins, Baltimore, Maryland, 1992
(6) Stumpf P: Estrogen Replacement Therapy: current regimens, In Hormone Replacement Therapy, edited by D.P. Swartz, chapter 183, Williams and Wilkins,

(6) Stumpf P: Estrogen Replacement Therapy: current regimens, In Hormone Replacement Therapy, edited by D.P. Swartz, chapter 183, Williams and Wilkins, Baltimore, Maryland, 1992

(7) Follingstad, AH: Estriol, the forgotten estrogen? JAMA 239:29-30, 1978

(8) Tzingounis VA, et al: Estriol in the management of menopause, JAMA 239:1638-41, 1978

(9) Prior J.C: Progesterone as a bone-trophic hormone, Endocrine Rev., 11:386-398, 1990.

(10) McNeeley SG Jr., et al: Prevention of osteoporosis by medroxyprogesterone acetate in postmenopausal women, Int. J. Gynecol. Obstet., 34:253-56, 1991

(11) Hammar M et al: Does physical exercise influence the frequency of post-menopausal hot flushes, Acta Obstet. Gynecol. Scand., 69:409-12, 1990

(12) Mindell Earl: Earl Mindell's Soy Miracle, Fireside series, Simon & Schuster, New York, NY, 1995

(13) Murase Y and Iishima H: Clinical studies of oral administration of gamma oryzanol on climacteric complaints and it's syndrome, Obstet. Gynecol. Prac., 12:147-95, 1963

(14) Cristy CJ: Vitamin E in Menopause, Am. J. Obstet. & Gyn., 50:84-6, 1945

(15) Finkler RSL The effect of vitamin E in menopause, J. Clin. Endocrin. Metabol., 9:89-94, 1949

(16) Neilsen FH, et al: Effect of dietary boron on mineral, estrogen and testosterone metabolism in postmenopausal women, FASEB J., 1:39407, 1987

(17) Reid Ian R et al: Effect of calcium Supplementation on Bone Loss in Postmenopausal Women, New Engl. J. Med., 328:400-4, 1993

(18) Elghamry MI, et al: Biological activity of phytoestrogens, Planta Medica 13:353-7, 1965

(19) Kaldas, RS and Hughes, CC: reproductive and general metabolic effects of phytoestrogens in mammals, Reprod. Toxicol., 3:81-9, 1989

(20) Leung AY: Common Natural Ingredients Used in Food, Drugs, and cosmetics, John Wiley & Sons, New York, NY, 1980

(21) The Lawrence Review of Natural Products: Alfalfa, Pharmaceutical Associates Ltd., Levittown, Pennsylvania,, January 1986

(22) Duke JA: Handbook of Medicinal Herbs, CRC Press, Boca Raton, Florida, 1985

(23) The Lawrence Review of Natural Products: The Cohosh's, Pharmaceutical Information Associates Ltd., Levittown, Pennsylvania, 6:5, May 1985

(24) Albert-Puleo M: Fennel and anise as estrogenic agents, J. Enthnopharmacology 2:337-44, 1980

(25) Bohnert KJ and Kahn G: Phytotherapy in gynecology and obstetrics: Vitex agnus castus, Erfahrungshlk 494-502, 1990

(26) Weiss RF: Herbal Medicine, Beaconsfield Publishers Ltd., Beaconsfield, England, 1988

(27) Hikino H: Recent research on Oriental medicinal plants, Economic Medical Plant Research 1:53-85

CHAPTER 23

RELIEVING PREMENSTRUAL STRESS

Premenstrual syndrome (PMS) is the term used to describe the group of symptoms that occur prior to the onset of menstruation in the normal female menstrual cycle. PMS has been reported to affect 70 to 90% of the female population. Between 20 and 40% of females report some degree of temporary mental and physical dysfunction and 2 to 5% may be incapacitated. It has been estimated that 20 to 40% of all women seek professional help with PMS symptoms. PMS is cross-cultural and affects women of all races, socio-economic status and professions. Increased age seems to play a role in the development of symptoms with approximately 50% of women between the ages of 30 and 40 showing three or more signs of PMS. The risk of developing PMS seems to increase with certain events such as puberty, pregnancy, childbirth, tubal ligation, peri-menopause, use of oral contraceptives, hysterectomy and major life stresses.

The exact cause of PMS is unknown although a dysfunction involving the hypothalamus-pituitary-ovarian axes is believed to be involved. Current theories suggest that PMS is secondary to estrogen excess, progesterone deficiency, low progesterone to estrogen ratio, or a precipitous drop in progesterone levels. Vitamin B6 and magnesium deficiencies have been implicated as a cause of PMS. In addition, hypoglycemia (low blood sugar), psychomotor and stress related factors, and elevated prolactin levels have also been suggested to play a role in the development of PMS. The diagnosis of PMS is based upon the occurrence of psychologic and somatic symptoms in relationship to the normal female cycle. Typical symptoms of PMS include anxiety, irritability, mood swings, nervous tension, increased appetite, headache, fatigue, dizziness, palpitations, depression, crying, forgetfulness, confusion, insomnia, fluid retention, weight gain, swollen extremities, breast tenderness and abdominal bloating. Natural therapies provide effective relief for the symptoms of premenstrual syndrome.

DIET

Women who consume large amounts of caffeine are more likely to develop PMS compared to women who don't consume caffeine. Sixty-one percent of women who drank 4.5 to 15 caffeine-containing drinks per day experienced moderate to severe symptoms, while only 16% of women consuming no caffeine experienced moderate to severe symptoms. Caffeine intake should be reduced three to seven days prior to onset of symptoms. (1) Excess intake of refined carbohydrates and sugar is associated with PMS. (2) Refined sugar increases the urinary excretion of magnesium, a deficiency which may contribute to the development of PMS. (3) During the luteal phase, the second half of the normal 28 day female cycle, cells have an increased capacity to bind insulin which may be further modified by sugar intake. (4) Excess salt intake can aggravate PMS and can lead to weight gain, abdominal bloating, breast tenderness and swollen extremities. (5) Daily salt intake should be reduced to less than 3 grams per day. Impaired absorption of magnesium can lead to high calcium levels, a high calcium/magnesium ratio and development of PMS symptoms. Dairy products and calcium should be reduced appropriately. (6)

NUTRIENTS

Supplementation with Pyridoxine (Vitamin B6) significantly improves symptoms associated with PMS. (7) Pyridoxine supplementation may help normalize deficient intracellular magnesium levels and is a co-factor in fatty acid metabolism. (8) Seventy to 80% of 630 women taking 80 to 200 mg of B6 daily reported significant improvement in the symptoms of PMS. (9) There were no cases of neuropathy and side effects were minimal.

Vitamin A supplementation during the second half of the normal female cycle significantly improved symptoms associated with PMS. (10)

Vitamin E supplementation may also be beneficial in reducing the severity of symptoms associated with PMS. (11)

Magnesium deficiency has been correlated with the development and severity of PMS symptoms. (12) Deficiency of magnesium cause adrenal cortex growth, leading to elevated aldosterone levels and increased fluid volume. (13) Magnesium is also required for the conversion of linoleic acid to gamma-linoleic acid by the enzyme delta-6-desaturase. (14) Magnesium may reduce glucose induced insulin secretion. Magnesium deficiency caused depletion of the brain neurotransmitter, dopamine. (15) Supplementation with magnesium relieves PMS symptoms. (16)

A functional deficiency of essential fatty acids, either due to inadequate linoleic acid intake or absorption or failure of normal conversion of linoleic acid to GLA has been postulated to cause abnormal sensitivity to prolactin and lead to the development of PMS. (17) Evening primrose oil (EPO) an omega-6 fatty acid and a source of gamma linoleic acid may inhibit glucose induced insulin secretion. (18) Supplementation with Evening Primrose oil can reduce symptoms associated with PMS. (19)

BOTANICAL MEDICINES

Phytoestrogens are plant sources of estrogens and estrogen precursors. Phytoestrogens are found in many plants and this may explain why different plants were traditionally used in various female disorders, including menstrual disorders, menopause, and PMS. (20) Phytoestrogens are 1:400 as active as estrogens found in animal sources, but plant estrogens due exert biological activity nonetheless. In humans, estrogens are formed in the ovary, adrenal cortex and the testes. Estrogens are primarily responsible for the development of female secondary sex characteristics and during the female menstrual cycle, responsible for providing an environment suitable for fertilization, implantation and nutrition of the developing embryo. Phytoestrogens are a source of exogenous estrogen and compete for estrogen receptor binding sites on cells. (20) When estrogen levels are low, phytoestrogens can bind to cell receptors and exert some estrogenic activity. When estrogen levels are high, phytoestrogens compete with estrogen in the body for receptor binding sites and can displace endogenous estrogen and limit its effects. This can explain why certain plants have been traditionally used as female regulators or balancers, to decrease estrogen levels when they are high and to increase estrogen levels when they are low. There are various plant sources of phytoestrogens.

Unicorn Root (Aletris Farinosa) is a perennial herb used as a folk remedy by American Indians for a variety of complaints including female disorders. Unicorn root contains essential oils, a resin and a steroidal saponin, diosgenin, that exerts estrogenic activity. (21)

Blue Cohosh (Caulophyllum thalictroides) is a perennial herb with a thick crooked rhizome native to eastern North America and grows up to 1 meter in height. Chemical constituents of Blue Cohosh include alkaloids including methylcytisine and triterpene glycosides called caulosaponins. Methylcytisine is pharmacologically similar to nicotine and results in increased blood pressure and pulse, stimulation of the small intestine and hyperglycemia. It is 10 to 40 times less active than nicotine and about one-fortieth as toxic. Caulosaponins are uterine stimulants, that also induce blood vessel constriction on heart muscle. Researchers in India have found that low dose extracts of Caulophyllum given to rats inhibit ovulation and result in uterine changes that will inhibit implantation of the fertilized egg and may have contraceptive potential. Ingestion of Blue Cohosh can cause stomach upset and vomiting. (21,22)

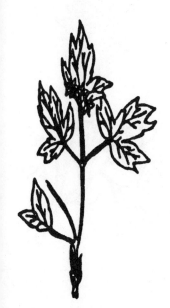

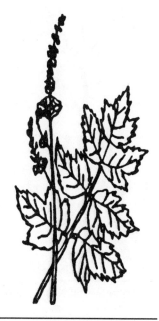

Blue Cohosh
(Caulophyllum thalictroides)

Black Cohosh
(Cimicifuga racemosa)

Black Cohosh (Cimicifuga racemosa) is a perennial herb that has been used medicinally by American Indians to cure dysmenorrhea. The root contains 15 to 20% of an amorphous resinous substance called cimicifugin and two triterpene glycosides, actein and cimigoside, that have been reported to exert estrogenic activity. Actein lowers blood pressure in rabbits and cats, but not dogs. The plant has also been reported to contain methylcytisine, a chemical similar to nicotine that produces increased blood pressure. Excess doses may produce nausea, vomiting and dizziness. (21)

Alfalfa (Medicago sativa) is a legume resembling clover that is cultivated throughout the world as animal forage. Alfalfa contains 2.0 to 3.0% steroidal saponins, flavonoids, coumarin derivatives and alkaloids. Coumarin derivatives and the flavone tricin produce estrogenic effects. Tricin inhibits smooth muscle contraction in the uterus and is an antioxidant. Alfalfa contains chemicals that produce a mild estrogen effect, which explains this plant's historical use for gynecological disorders. (21,23)

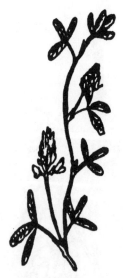

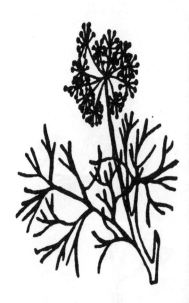

Alfalfa (Medicago sativa)   Fennel (Foeniculum vulgare)

Fennel (Foeniculum vulgare) is an aromatic herb native to southern Europe and Asia minor and is cultivated throughout North America. The name foeniculum is derived from the latin word meaning fragrant. Fennel seeds contain 3 to 6% of an essential oil and up to 20% fixed oil which accounts for its characteristic odor. Fennel has been reported to increase milk secretion, promote menstruation, facilitate birth, ease the female climacteric and increase libido. The estrogenic component of fennel is believed to be anethole and anethole polymers. Ingestion of the volatile oil fraction of fennel can produce nausea, vomiting and contact dermatitis. (24)

Chaste tree (Vitex agnus castus) is a plant native to the Mediterranean and central Asia. As it name suggests it was once used to suppress libido. Fruit of this plant has been used medicinally. The fruit contains volatile oils to which they attribute a pleasant peppermint-like smell. The volatile oil constituents of Vitex act upon the hypothalamus in the brain. It causes an increase in leutinizing hormone (LH) production and a decrease in follicle stimulating hormone (FSH) production. As a result there is an increase in production of progesterone with a corresponding decrease in estrogen. (25)

Dong quai (Angelica sinensis) is a stout biennial or perennial herb growing up to 2 meters high and is native to mainland China. Angelica sinensis has been used for thousands of years in oriental medicine in the treatment of various female disorders and is second in reputation to ginseng. The root and rhizome contains 0.3 to 1.0% volatile oil and 0.2% coumarin derivatives. The coumarin derivatives are believed to be responsible for pharmacologic effects of this plant. Angelica has demonstrated analgesic, anti-inflammatory, uterine smooth muscle relaxing, estrogenic and immuno-modulating activity. Few adverse side effects have been reported including contact dermatitis, stomach upset, muscle cramping and photosensitivity. (21,26)

RECOMMENDATIONS: Daily unless otherwise stated

Vitamin B6..50-100 mg
Vitamin A..50,000-100,000 IU
Vitamin E...300-600 IU
Magnesium..400-800 mg
Omega-6 Oil (Evening primrose oil)................500-1500 mg
Aletris farinosa (4:1)..100-200 mg
Caulophyllum thalictroides (4:1)..........................200-300 mg
Cimicifuga racemosa (4:1)................................200-300 mg

Medicago sativa (4:1)...500-1000 mg
Foeniculum vulgare (6:1)...75-100 mg
Vitex agnus castus...200-300 mg
Angelica sinensis (4:1)..500-1000 mg

REFERENCES

(1) Rossignol AM: Caffeine-containing beverages and premenstrual syndrome in young women. Am. J. Public Health 75(11):1335-37, 1985
(2) Goei GS et al: Dietary patterns of patients with premenstrual tension. J. Applied Nutr. 34(1):4-11, 1982
(3) Seelig M. Human requirements of magnesium: Factors that increase need in Durlach J, Ed. First Int. Sympos. on Magnesium Deficiency in Human Pathology. Paris, Springer, Verlag, p. 11, 1971
(4) Muggeo M et al: Change in affinity of insulin receptors following oral glucose in normal adults. J. Clin. Endocrinol. Metabol. 44:1206-9, 1977
(5) Ferrannini E et al: Sodium elevates the plasma glucose response to glucose ingestion in man. J. Clin. Endocrinol. Metab. 54:455, 1982
(6) Abraham GE: Magnesium deficiency in premenstrual tension. Magnesium Bulletin 1:68-73, 1982
(7) Abraham GE: personal communication reported in Piesse JW. Nutrition factors in the premenstrual syndrome. Int. Clin. Nutr. Rev. 4(2):54-81, 1984
(8) Abraham GE et al: Effect of vitamin B6 on plasma and red blood cell magnesium levels in premenopausal women. Ann. Clin. Lab Sci. 11(4):333-36, 1981
(9) Williams MJ et al: Controlled trial of pyridoxine in the premenstrual syndrome. J. Int. Med. Res. 13:174-79. 1985
(10) Block E: The use of vitamin A in premenstrual tension. Acta Obst. Gynec. Scand. 39:586-92, 1960(11) London RS et al: J. Am. Coll. Nutr. 3(4):351-6, 1984
(12) Abraham GE et al: Serum and red cell magnesium levels in patients with premenstrual tension. Am. J. Clin. Nutr. 34:1264-66, 1981
(13) Horton R et al: Effect of aldosterone on the metabolism of magnesium. J. Clin. Endocrinol. 22:1187, 1962
(14) Cunane SC et al: Parenteral linoleic and gamma-linoleic acids ameliorate the gross effects of zinc deficiency. Proc. Soc. Exp. Biol & Med. 164:583, 1980
(15) Curry DL et al: Magnesium modulation of glucose-induced insulin secretion by the perfused rat pancreas. Endocrinolgy 101:203, 1977
(16) Nicholas A: Traitement du syndrome premenstruel et de la dysmenorrhee par l'ion magnesium. in Durlach J, Ed. First Int. sympos. on Magnesium Deficiency in Human Pathology. Paris, Springer, Verlag, pp. 261-3, 1973
(17) Horrobin DF: The role of essential fatty acids and prostaglandins in the premenstrual syndrome. J. Reprod. Med. 28(7):465-68, 1983
(18) Gugliano D et al: Prostaglandin E1 inhibits glucose-induced insulin secretion in man. Prostaglandins Med. 48:302, 1979

(19) Brush MG: Evening primrose oil in the treatment of the premenstrual syndrome. Clinical Uses of Essential Fatty Acids. Montreal, Eden Press, pp. 155-62, 1982

(20) Elghamry MI et al: Biological activity of phytoestrogens. Planta Medica 13:353-7. 1965

(21) Leung AY: Common Natural Ingredients Used in Food, Drugs, and Cosmetics, John Wiley & Sons, New York, NY, 1980

(22) The Lawrence Review of Natural Products: The Cohosh's. Pharmaceutical Information Associates, Ltd. Levittown, Pennsylvania, 6:5, May 1985

(23) The Lawrence Review of Natural Products: Alfalfa. Pharmaceutical Information Associates, Ltd. Levittown, Pennsylvania, January 1986

(24) Albert-Puleo M: Fennel and anise as estrogenic agents. J. Ethnopharmacology 2:337-44, 1980

(25) Weiss RF: Herbal Medicine. Beaconsfield Publishers Ltd. Beaconsfield, England, 1988

(26) Hikino H: Recent research on Oriental medicinal plants. Economic Medical Plant Research 1:53-85, 1985

CHAPTER 24

TONIC FOR FATIGUE AND LETHARGY

Fatigue is a generalized feeling of tiredness or exhaustion and involves loss of power or capacity to respond to stimulation. Fatigue is a normal reaction to physical exertion, emotional strain or lack of sleep and is experienced by all of us at one time or another. Fatigue is usually short lived and responds to rest, relaxation, a hearty meal and a good night's sleep. However, if fatigue becomes persistent and does not respond to rest, then a more serious underlying disorder is indicated. Many diseases are capable of producing persistent fatigue including cancer and heart disease. A proper medical workup is required to diagnose the cause of persistent fatigue. Fatigue, sore throat, lymph node enlargement and muscle aches are common symptoms used to describe a term called chronic fatigue syndrome.

This illness is chronic and recurrent, as its name suggests and can last from a few months to a few years. Chronic Fatigue Syndrome affects twice as many females as males and is more common in young and middle aged adults. The illness may follow a viral infection, but may also appear spontaneously. The onset of the syndrome typically seems to be in late adolescence or young adulthood, although it may occur earlier or later. Although fatigue is common among the elderly, chronic fatigue syndrome is not. There is no typical patient profile in individuals with this illness. CFS can affect young college students, housewives, construction workers and professionals such as doctors and lawyers.

The conventional medical establishment continues to fail to recognize CFS as a genuine illness. Subsequently, few physicians are sympathetic and understanding to individuals suffering from chronic fatigue of unknown origin. New research and clinical practice confirm that CFS is a real illness with profound impact on those individuals afflicted with it. Natural therapies including diet and nutritional supplementation and herbal medicine can help improve this condition.

LIFESTYLE

There is a significant relationship between psychological state and Chronic Fatigue Syndrome. Psychological and stress-related factors are associated with the onset and severity of Chronic Fatigue Syndrome. Individuals should be encouraged to evaluate the stressors in their life and reduce the demands they make on themselves and others. Illness such as Chronic Fatigue Syndrome, may be a time for introspection and a time for an individual to become aware and sensitive to their psyche and body. Stress reduction techniques such as relaxation, deep breathing, meditation, visualization and hypnosis should be explored. Supportive therapy and counselling may be beneficial. (1)

Regular exercise, at least three to four times a week, is an important means of stress reduction and makes the body feel better. There is also mounting evidence that moderate exercise can stimulate immune function. Although individuals with chronic fatigue may be too tired to exercise, a conscious effort to walk outdoors on a regular basis should be encouraged. A brisk walk, swimming, cycling, or other aerobic exercises are strongly recommended. (1)

DIET

Diet plays a very important role in all aspects of human physiology including energy level and immune function. A poor diet high in refined carbohydrates, fats and processed foods is associated with decreased energy levels. A liberal consumption of water is necessary for the body to run efficiently and six to eight glasses of water per day is recommended. Manipulation of dietary factors has been shown to optimize immune function. Adequate dietary protein is necessary for proper immune function. Excessive intake of fats including cholesterol and polyunsaturated fats is associated with immune depression. Sugar impairs all aspects of immune function and should be avoided. A well balanced diet emphasizing whole, unprocessed and unrefined foods is strongly recommended. Complex carbohydrates, fruits and vegetables and fiber should be increased. The diet should include a wide variety of foods to maintain proper nutrition and prevent nutritional deficiencies. (2,3)

NUTRIENTS

A reduced intake of B-complex vitamins can lead to decreased endurance and increased fatigability. Supplementation with B-complex vitamins can improve performance in those individuals whose intake is less than 35-45% of the RDA. (4,5)

Folic acid deficiency is associated with fatigability and supplementation can prevent ease of fatigue. (5)

Pantothenic acid (Vitamin B5) deficiency is associated with tiredness, insomnia, sullenness and depression and supplementation can help improve these symptoms. (6)

Pyridoxine (Vitamin B6) supplementation helps maintain muscle contractions longer when it was added to a normal diet. (7)

Vitamin B12 supplementation helps to decrease fatigue and improves general well being. Although the exact mechanism of action is not known, functions of this vitamin include maturation of red blood cells, genetic DNA production and nerve function. (8)

Reduced consumption of Vitamin C is associated with increased fatigability and other related symptoms. Vitamin C is also widely used for its immune supporting and antiviral activity. (9)

Iron is intimately associated with production of red blood cells and the oxygen carrying capacity of blood. Iron deficiency is associated with reduced work capacity and increased onset of fatigue. Iron supplementation to treat anemia can improve work capacity and reduce fatigability. (10)

Magnesium is required for energy production and for muscle contraction. Magnesium deficiency results in irritability of the nervous system, fatigue, muscle spasms, convulsions, tremors, depression and psychotic behavior. Stress, anxiety and nervousness alone can lead to magnesium deficiency. Individuals with Chronic Fatigue Syndrome have low red blood cell magnesium levels and those treated with magnesium alone reported significant improvement in overall well being and reduced fatigue. Magnesium supplementation improves energy status and should be taken by all individuals suffering from chronic fatigue. (11)

Potassium is important in regulating acid-base balance in the body and is involved in nerve function and muscle contraction. Potassium deficiency is associated with chronic muscle weakness and chronic tiredness. Potassium supplementation can improve the symptoms of deficiency. (12)

Zinc supplementation can improve muscle strength and endurance in some individuals. (13)

Liver extract preparations provide a high dose of B-complex vitamins, iron and proteins that display immune stimulating qualities. Liver extract preparations have been used successfully to treat individuals with Chronic Fatigue Syndrome. (14)

The thymus is a small gland lying beneath the sternum in the upper chest that plays an important role in immune development. The thymus reaches its maximum development during puberty and continues to play an important role in immune function throughout life. The thymus gland is responsible for the maturation of a type of white blood cell called a T-lymphocyte (T denoting thymus). The thymus produces mature lymphocytes that are active in protecting the body from foreign invaders that might otherwise cause infection. Abnormal T-lymphocyte counts are the hallmark of Chronic Fatigue Syndrome. Thymus gland preparations have been used to increase immune response to a number of diseases including Chronic Fatigue Syndrome. (15)

OTHER FACTORS

Food and environmental allergies and sensitivities have been associated with increased fatigability, loss of energy and endurance, irritability, headache and depression. Food and environmental allergies and sensitivities should be considered in the evaluation of all individuals suffering from Chronic Fatigue Syndrome. (16)

Hypoglycemia (low blood sugar) should be considered with episodic fatigue, weakness and apathy that is relieved shortly after eating. (17)

BOTANICAL MEDICINES

Siberian ginseng (Eleutherococcus senticosus) is a perennial shrub that is indigenous to certain parts of eastern Russia, China and Korea. Eleutherococcus is a member of the Aralaceae family; the same family as Panax ginseng. Unlike the smaller Panax species, Eleutherococcus commonly attains a height of two to three metres and rarely to five metres. Eleuthercoccus grows at elevations up to 800 metres or more above sea level in forests of broad leaf trees including spruce and cedar. The root of this plant is used in herbal medicine and has been popularized as a substitute for Panax ginseng. (18,19)

In 1855, Russian scientists discovered Eleutherococcus along the shores of Amur River and named the plant Eleutherococcus senticosus meaning "free -berried thorny shrub." It wasn't till the 1950's that Russian scientists rediscovered the plant in their search for a suitable and inexpensive alternative to Panax ginseng. The plant was popularized as a stimulating and rejuvenating herb. The Soviet pharmacologists I. I. Brekhman and I.V. Dardymov conducted extensive research on the pharmacological properties of a 33% alcoholic extract of the plant. (18,19)

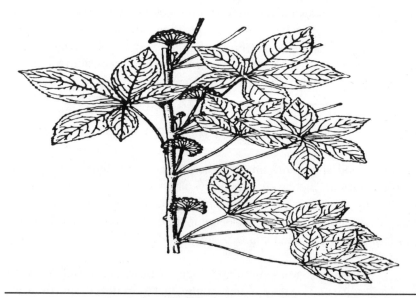

Siberian ginseng (Eleutherococcus senticosus)

Active ingredients in siberian ginseng are believed to be a group of related chemicals called eleutherosides. At least seven different eleutherosides, termed eleutherosides A to G, have been isolated from the roots of siberian ginseng. Eleutherosides A to G occur in the roots of this plant in the following ratio of 8:30:10:12:4:2:1. Total eleutheroside content of the root has been determined to be in the range 0.6 to 0.9% and of the stem in the range of 0.6 to 1.5%. The chemical composition of the root varies with the season. The roots show maximum active ingredients in October while the levels decrease in July. Thin layer chromatography has shown that the elutherosides are not present in the roots of panax or korean red ginseng. While there are structural similarities between the compounds in the two ginseng species they are chemically distinct and unique. (18,19,20)

Eleutherococcus has demonstrated significant anti-stress activity. It is believed that eleutherosides from siberian ginseng bind to hormone receptors in the body. They specifically bin to progestin, minerallocorticoid and glucocorticoid receptors. This may explain the glucocorticoid activity of Eleutherococcus. Eleutherosides stimulate the pituitary gland in the brain to produce ACTH (Adrenocorticotropic hormone) an adrenal gland stimulating hormone. ACTH travels via the bloodstream to the adrenal glands and stimulates the production of glucocorticoids. Glucocorticoids including cortisol, cortisone and hydrocortisone are a group of steroidal hormones that exert many physiologic effects on the body. They are widely known for the anti-inflammatory and anti-stress effects. In addition, they promote the breakdown of fats and triglycerides and increase the breakdown of protein and amino acids. Collectively these actions raise blood sugar levels and the ability of blood glucose to cells throughout the body. Eleutherococcus extracts reduced the increase in weight of adrenal glands in response to prolonged stress and decreased blood levels of vitamin C and cholesterol. Futhermore, administration of Eleutherococcus to physiologically stressed animals prevented thymus gland atrophy and lymphatic involution. (20,22)

Administration of Eleutherococcus extracts stimulates DNA synthesis and increases the rate of growth and protein formation in frogs and sea urchin embryos. Oral administration of Eleutherococcus to dogs increased the conditioned response to stimuli. Administration to mice increased aerobic swimming performance in mice. (18)

Eleutherococcus has demonstrated a normalizing effect on blood pressure in both hypertension and hypotension. Eleutherococcus decreases high blood pressure through improvement of atherosclerosis and reduction in the production of cholesterol in the liver. Eleutherococcus also decreased low blood pressure. In hypotensive children between seven and ten years of age, an extract of Eleutherococcus improved subjective signs of low blood pressure and raised both systolic and diastolic pressure. (18)

Eleutherococcus has been used to help normalize blood sugar levels in diabetics. Eleuthero extracts have been reported to reduce blood sugar levels by enhancing the synthesis of glycogen and high energy phosphate molecules. Eleutherococcus reduces blood sugar in alimentary and adrenal hyperglycemia and increases blood sugar levels in insulin-induced hypoglycemia. Furthermore, Eleutherococcus stimulates the adrenal glands to produce glucocorticoid hormone which directly affect blood sugar levels. (18)

Eleutherococcus has displayed immune stimulating activity. Eleuthero reduces susceptibility and increases resistance to viral infection in animal experiments. In one study, 36 healthy volunteers received an alcoholic extract of eleutherococcus in the form of an injection three times per day for four weeks. Drastic increases in the numbers of immunocompetent cells and particularly T-cells were observed. The increase was most marked for helper/inducer cells, although cytotoxic and natural killer cells were also increased. A general enhancement of cell-mediated immunity was evident. (18)

Eleutherococcus has also demonstrated radioprotective effects to cells following exposure to ionizing radiation. Eleutherococcus increased resistance to the ionizing radiation and the effects was indirect due to an alteration of cell susceptibility rather than affecting DNA repair processes. Russian scientists have reported a doubling and tripling of survival time of mice treated with Eleutherococcus during exposure to chronic radiation of up to 7000 rads and after acute radiation to 800 rads. (25)

Eleutherococcus extracts have also displayed anti-proliferative effects against certain types of cancer cells. Oral administration of Eleutherococcus extracts to rodents has been reported to delay tumour formation, prevent or delay metastasis, prevent or delay spontaneous mammary tumour or spontaneous induction of leukemia. Furthermore, Eleutherococcus has demonstrated anti-toxic effects to various toxic substances including cytarabine and N-6-adenosine in partially hepatectomized animals. This suggests that addition of the extracts to anti-cancer regimes might make possible the reductions of dosed of these toxic substances. (18,20,22)

In clinical studies, Eleutherococcus root extracts we administered orally to 2100 human subjects. These studies were designed to measure the ability of humans to withstand adverse reactions to various external stimuli including heat, noise, motion, workload increase, exercise, decompression, mental activity and to work under stressed conditions and athletic performance. Both male and female subjects ranged in age from 19 to 72 years. They received 2.0 to 16.0 millilitres of a 33% ethanolic extract of siberian ginseng root for up to sixty consecutive days. Eleuthercoccus extracts provided significant anti-stress activity and improved all reactions to the various stimuli. (23) In another study a 23.3% increase in total work capacity versus 7.5 % increase in work capacity with placebo in human subjects. Significant improvement in oxygen uptake and maximum oxygen pulse was observed in the eleutherococcus treated group. Researchers confirmed some of the uses of siberian ginseng extract as and ergogenic aid in athletes. A 33% ethanolic extract was approved by the Pharmacologic Committee of the U.S.S.R.Ministry of Health for human use in 1962. (24) In 1976 it was estimated that there were more than three million regular users in the former Soviet Union. Eleutherococcus was widely promoted as an adaptogen to help the body deal with stress and improve energy and vitality.

Siberian ginseng is innocuous and few side effects have been reported. Occasional adverse effects include allergic reaction, stomach upset, insomnia and irritability. No long term toxicity has been reported and the LD50 of the 33% ethanolic extract is 14.5 ml/kg in mice and greater than 20.0 ml/kg in rats. Use of siberian ginseng during pregnancy is discouraged. (18,19,21)

The ancient Chinese used ginseng for thousands of years for it's tonifying and tranquilizing effects on the human body. Ginseng literally means "essence of man" and belongs to the Araliaceae family. The are several different species of ginseng that have been used medicinally including Panax ginseng which grows in northern China otherwise known as chinese ginseng or in Korea otherwise known as Korean ginseng. Panax ginseng is a small, woody perennial plant that grows in swampy, damp forests. Panax ginseng is further classified as white or red ginseng. White ginseng is simply the dried root while red ginseng is the root steamed in caramel or other dye. In addition to Panax there are several other species of related ginseng including Japanese ginseng (Panax japonicus), San-chi ginseng (Panax notoginseng), Himalayan ginseng (Panax pseudoginseng) and American ginseng (Panax quinquefolium). (18,19,21)

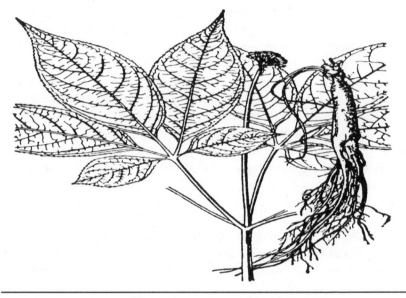

Korean ginseng (Panax ginseng)

Ginseng is perhaps the most studied of the herbal medicines throughout the world. Biochemical analysis has identified over thirty different triterpenoid glycosides that have been isolated from the roots of the various species. These triterpenoid glycosides are steroidal molecules that are believed to be the primary active ingredients in ginseng root. These triterpenoid glycosides have been further classified into three related groups. Oleanolic acid derivatives have been designated ginsenoside Ro. Protopanaxadiol derivatives have been designated ginsenoside fractions Rb1 to Rd. Protopanaxatriol derivatives have been designated ginsenoside fractions Re to Rg2. Researchers believe that these ginsenosides fractions are responsible for the purported medicinal effects of ginseng. Other constituents include steroidal compounds, carbohydrates, starch, vitamin B and C, choline, peptides, amino acids and trace minerals such as iron, zinc copper, manganese, vanadium and germanium. (18,19,26)

The triperpenoid content of ginseng root is usually to 2.0 to 5.0% of the dry weight of the root. The different species of ginseng differ with respect to the relative proportions of the different triterpenoid glycosides. Panax ginseng contains a high content of ginsenosides Rb1, Rb2, Rc, Re and Rg1. In contrast American ginseng contains only significant amounts of Rb1 and Re. With these different triterpenoid proportions in mind it should be noted that Panax ginseng is used as a nervous system stimulant and adaptogen for stress. American ginseng contains fewer stimulating glycosides and is primarily noted for it's nervous system depressant activity. (18,26)

The pharmacologic properties of the Rb1 and Rg1 triterpenoid fractions of panax ginseng have been explored in detail by Chinese, Japanese and European researchers. The Rb1 fraction exerts central nervous system depressant activity, anti-psychotic and anti-ulcer activity. In contrasts the Rg1 fraction exerts central nervous system stimulant activity. This is particularly interesting when comparing the activity of different ginseng preparation that contain different ginsenoside content. Siberian ginseng contains a higher concentration of Rb1 ginsenoside while chinese ginseng typically contains a higher concentration of Rg1 ginsenoside. American ginseng contains very few ginsenoside with central nervous system stimulating properties. It is typically recommended for the treatment of insomnia, nervousness, indigestion and toothaches. Panax ginseng can produce nervous system stimulant and depressant actions based on the respective concentrations of different ginsenosides. It is worthwhile to note that panax ginseng is recommended to be an adaptogen or supplement that helps the body deal with stress. It's action is non-specific and it can exert a calming effect or a stimulating effect depending on the state of the nervous system. (18,26,27)

The ginsenoside Rg1 stimulates the pituitary gland to produce adrenocorticotropic hormone or ACTH. (27) ACTH stimulates the adrenal glands to produce a group of adrenal gland hormones called glucocorticoid.   Glucocorticoids include cortisol, cortisone and hydrocortisone. Endogenous cortisol has many effects throughout the body including promoting the body's ability to respond to long term stress. Cortisol acts on the liver and stimulates the production of glucose, increases the breakdown of fats and fatty acids and increases the breakdown of protein into amino acids. All these actions collectively increase the supply of glucose and energy producing molecules to produce energy for muscles and the nervous system. (28)

Administration of panax ginseng extracts causes a decrease in an enzyme called alpha-hydroxybutyrate dehydrogenase. This enzyme causes a consequent decrease in lactic acid production in muscle tissue. Exercise physiologists believe that a buildup of lactic acid in muscle tissue is responsible for the typical muscle fatigue that we experience with strenuous physical exercise. Panax ginseng has obvious prophylactic benefit for athletes. (29)

Recent research indicates that ginseng lowers total cholesterol levels and has an anti-atherosclerotic effect. Panax ginseng decreased both total cholesterol and low density lipoprotein (LDL) cholesterol while increasing high density lipoprotein (HDL) levels. Panax ginseng also stimulates an enzyme called lipoprotein lipase which hydrolyzes intravascular chylomicrons and prevents atheroma formation. (29)

Ginseng confer some resistance to the damaging effects of radiation. Animal studies indicate that a dose dependent quantity of ginseng root prior to radiation exposure increases survival time of tested animals. In addition blood cell levels, increased DNA content and decreased hemorrhaging was noted. (30) Ginseng potentiates an increase in DNA and protein synthesis in rapidly dividing cells such as bone marrow, germ cells and liver cells. (31)

The normal effects of aging increase the free radical damage on the human body. Free radicals are highly reactive unpaired electrons that react with normal body cells. Ginseng prevents free radical damage to fatty membranes of cells and the generation of damaging peroxides within cells. Research indicates that panax ginseng possesses significant antioxidant ability and holds promise as a potent antioxidant. Also in animal and in vitro experiments panax ginseng has shown anti-neoplastic effects and has inhibited the growth of cancerous tissue in certain types of cancer including leukemia, lung adenoma and hepatomas of the liver. (25,30)

Some research indicates the panax ginseng influences the immune system. Antiviral effects to certain viruses has been demonstrated as well as delayed hypersensitivity to certain viruses. Panax ginseng supplementation helped to raise antibody levels and boosted certain aspects of cell mediated immunity. (30)

Clinical studies support the anti-stress and anti-fatigue qualities of panax ginseng. Oxygen absorption capacity measured as V02 maximum which is an index of sustained work capacity. Ginseng decreases lactic acid production which decreases muscle fatigability. Ginseng decreases heart rate and helps to stabilize blood sugar levels. Ginseng increases physical as well mental functioning. It increases mental alertness, reaction time and power of concentration. (24,32)

The therapeutic effects of panax ginseng are directly related to the ginsenoside content of the root of the plant. This should be reflected in the dosage of the plant ingested. Current research indicates the optimal dosage would be 25 milligrams of the ginseng glycoside Rg1 for it's stimulating and tonifying effects. The Rg1 fraction contained in many commercial products varies considerably. The Rg1 concentration of ginseng root varies from 0% to 18% of the dry weight of the root in some concentrated extracts. Average crude products have a ginsenoside content between 0.5 to 5.0%. As an example of a ginseng preparation that contains 5.0% Rg1 content you would need 500 milligrams of crude plant to give you a daily dosage of 25 milligrams Rg1 ginsenoside. (18,26)

RECOMMENDATIONS: Daily unless otherwise stated

B-complex..50-100 mg
Folic acid...400-800 mcg
Pantothenic Acid (Vitamin B5)..............................500-1500 mg
Pyridoxine (Vitamin B6)...25-50 mg
Vitamin B12...100-200 mcg
Vitamin C..1000-3000 mg
Iron...10-25mg
Magnesium...400-800 mg
Potassium...1000-2000 mg
Zinc...25-50 mg
Liver Extract...1000-2000 mg

Eleutherococcus senticosus (4:1)..500-1000 mg
Panax ginseng (4:1)..500-1000 mg

REFERENCES

(1) Werbach MR: Nutritional Influences of Illness Keats Publishing Inc. New Canaan, Conneticut, 1987

(2) Guyton AC: Textbook of Medical Physiology 7th edition, WB Saunders Company, Philadelphia, Penn., 1986

(3) Holmes GP et al: Chronic Fatigue Syndrome: A Working Case Definition. Annals of Internal Medicine. 108: 387-389, 1988

(4) Conman LC: Effects of specific nutrients on the immune response. Med. Clin. North Am. 69(4):759-91, 1985

(5) van der Beek EJ: Vitamins and endurance training: Food for running or faddish claims? Sports Med. 2(3):175-97, 1985

(6) Clin. Psychiat. News, April 1976

(7) Richardson JH et al: The effect of B6 on muscle fatigue. J. Sports Med. Phys. Fitness 21(2):119-21, 1981

(8) Ellis FR et al: A pilot study of vitamin B12 in the treatment of tiredness. Brit. J. Nutr. 30:277-83, 1973

(9) Cheraskin E et al: Daily vitamin C consumption and fatigability. J. Am. Geriat. Soc. 24(3):136-37, 1976

(10) Gardner GW et al: Physical work capacity and metabolic stress in subjects with iron deficiency anemia. Am. J. Clin. Nutr. 30(6):910-917, 1977

(11) Cox IM et al: Red blood cell magnesium and chronic fatigue syndrome. Lancet 337:757-60, 1991

(12) Snively WD et al: Minnesota Medicine, June 1965

(13) Krotkiewski M et al: Zinc and muscle strength and endurance. Acta Physiol. Scand. 116(3):309-11, 1982

(14) Steinbach TL et al: Treatment of CFIDS with Kutapressin: Chronic Fatigue and Immune Dysfunction, Spring/Summer pp. 25-30, 1990

(15) Cazzola P et al: In vivo modulating effect of calf thymus acid lysate on human T lymphocyte subsets and CD4+/CD8+ ratio in the course of different diseases. Curr. Ther. Res. 42:1011-17, 1987

(16) Crook WG: Can Your Child Read? Is He Hyperactive? Jackson, Professional Books, 1977

(17) Breneman JC: Basics of Food Allergy. Springfield Illinois, Charles D. Thomas, 1978

(18) Pizzorno JE and Murray MT: A Textbook of Natural Medicine. JBC Publications, Seattle, Washington, 1985

(19) Leung AY: Encyclopedia of Common Natural Ingredients Used in Food, Drugs and Cosmetics. John Wiley & Sons, New York, NY 1980. pp 186-9

(20) Farnsworth NR et al: Siberian ginseng (Eleutherococcus senticosus): Current status as an adaptogen. Econ Med Plant Res. 1:156-215, 1985

(21) Duke JA: Handbook of Medicinal Herbs. CRC Presss, Boca Raton, FL, 1985, pp 337-8

(22) Brekhman II and Dardymov IV: New substances of plant origin which increase nonspecific resistance. Ann Rev Pharmacol. 9:419-30, 1969

(23) Katsumi Asano et al: Effect of Eleutherococcus senticosus on Human Physical Working Capacity. Planta Med. no.3 June 1985, pp 175-9

(24) McNaughton Lars et al: A comparison of Chinese and Russian Ginseng as ergogenic aids to improve various facets of physical fitness. Int Clin Nutr Rev. 1989 Vol. 9 No. 1, pp 32-5

(25) Ben-Hur E and Fulder S: Effect of P. ginseng saponins and Eleutherococcus s. on survival of cultured mammalian cells after ionizing radiation. Am J Chin Med 9:48-56, 1981

(26) Shibata S et al: Chemistry and pharmacology of Panax. Economic and Medicinal research 1:217-84, 1985

(27) Pekov W: The mechanism of action of P. ginseng. C.A. Meyer. Arzneim Forsch. 9:305-11, 1959

(28) Fulder SJ: Ginseng and the hypothalamic control of stress. Am J Chin Med. 9:112-8, 1981

(29) Avakia EV and Evonuk E: Effects of Panax ginseng extract on tissue glycogen and adrenal cholesterol depletion during prolonged exercise. Planat Med 36:43-8, 1979

(30) Singh SKF et al: Immunomodulatory activity of Panax ginseng extract. Planta Medica 51: 462-5, 1984

(31) Yamamoto M et al: Stimulatory effect of P. ginseng principles on DNA and protein synthesis. Arzneim Forsch 27:1404-5, 1977

(32) Hallstrom C et al: Effect of ginseng on the performance of nurses on night duty. Comp Med East & West, 6:277-82, 1982

CHAPTER 25

TREATMENT FOR INSOMNIA

Insomnia is defined as difficulty falling asleep or difficulty maintaining sleep with frequent or early awakenings. Fifteen to 25% of the population admit to varying degrees of insomnia and about 10% resort to chemical alternatives to treat their insomnia. Six to ten million people in North America use sedative-hypnotics or sleeping pills to treat insomnia. Common causes of insomnia include anxiety, tension, psychological stress, pain, environmental change, caffeine, alcohol, drugs and hypoglycemia. Safe, natural alternatives are available to treat insomnia that are effective and have only minimal side effects.

DIET

All caffeine sources should be eliminated. Coffee, tea, colas, chocolate and certain caffeine containing analgesics should be eliminated from the diet. The relative risk of insomnia for people consuming one to three cups of coffee a day (240 to 720 mg of caffeine) is 1.4 times for both males and females. (1) Low alcohol consumption may be beneficial while higher doses of alcohol may disrupt normal sleeping patterns. (2)

NUTRIENTS

Supplementation with various nutrients may be beneficial in many cases of insomnia. Myo-inositol may produce a calming effect and was found to alter EEG patterns similar to many anti-anxiety drugs. (3) Niacinamide is helpful for those who have difficulty maintaining sleep and who are often interrupted by frequent or early awakenings. Niacinamide was found to produce anti-conflict, anti-aggressive, muscle relaxant and hypnotic actions comparable to the action of minor tranquilizers. (4) L-Tryptophan, a precursor to the brain neurotransmitter serotonin, plays an important role in the induction and the maintenance of sleep. One gram of L-Tryptophan 30 to 60 minutes before bedtime decreases the time needed for the onset of sleep and increases the duration of sleep. Higher doses of L-Tryptophan up to 10 to 15 grams a day did not distort sleep patterns and had negligible level of side effects. Protein intake should be avoided for 90 minutes before and after administration of L-Tryptophan, as L-Tryptophan is an amino acid and other amino acids from protein may compete for the same receptor for uptake to the brain. (5)

BOTANICAL MEDICINES

Hops (Humulus lupulus) is a perennial climbing plant used extensively in the brewing industry. Hops has been used ever since the middle ages to treat nervousness, insomnia and irritability. Hops contains 0.3 to 1.0% volatile oil and up to 30% bitter resins known as humulone. (6) Hops also contains a volatile alcohol known only as 2-Methyl-3-butene-2-ol which is responsible for the sedative action of hops. After drying of the hops, the concentrations of this compound increases up to 0.15%. (7)

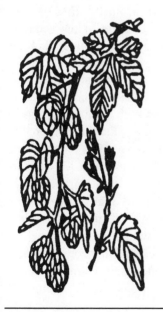 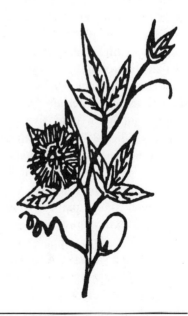

Hops (Humulus lupulus)   Passionflower (Passiflora incarnata)

Passion flower (Passiflora incarnata) is a perennial vine native to the southern United States. Passion flower contains 0.01 to 0.09% indole alkaloids and free flavonoids. Leaves have the highest alkaloid content and fruit rinds contain up to 0.25% alkaloids. (6) Both the alkaloids and the flavonoids are responsible for the sedative action of Passion flower. The harmala alkaloids have been found to inhibit monamine oxidase and related enzymes in the brain which inhibits breakdown of neurotransmitters in the central nervous system. Harmine was earlier known as "telepathine" and was used in World War II as "truth serum" to induce a relaxed, contemplative state in prisoners when under interrogation. (8)

Valerian (Valerian officinalis) is a perennial herb that grows up to 1.5 meters in height and is native to the temperate zones of North America, Europe and Asia. Valerian has a very distinctive, strong odor. (6) Valerian has been called "the valium of the 19th century" and has been widely used as a sedative-hypnotic for hundreds of years. Valerian contains a group of iridoid esters known as valepotriates. Valepotriates are present in all parts of the plant, but are found in highest concentration in the root, ranging from 0.1 to 2.0% dry weight. (9) Early investigators believed that the valepotriates were exclusively responsible for the sedative action of this plant. However, current research indicates that a volatile oil, ranging from 0.5 to 2.0% dry weight of the plant, is responsible in part for some of the sedative actions of this plant. Other constituents of Valerian include alkaloids which are present in smaller amounts and may contribute to the sedative action of the plant. The whole plant is more effective than the isolated constituents. Valerian has antispasmodic, muscle-relaxant, CNS-depressant and hypotensive effects. Studies on both animal and human models indicate that Valerian reduces sleep latency; the time required to fall asleep, increases the quality of sleep and has no effect on nocturnal movement. When 400 mg of Valerian extract was given to 128 patients in a double blind study, it was reported that patients significantly improved sleep quality. Similar results showed that 450 mg of a Valerian extract produced the same results as 900 mg of the same extract. Valerian compares favorably with synthetic sedatives such as Valium and Xanax. And unlike barbiturates and benzodiazepenes, Valerian does not cause addiction and dependence. In Germany, many doctors routinely prescribe Valerian preparations, where doctors in North America might resort to Valium and Xanax. Adverse effects to chronic Valerian use include headaches, irritability, drowsiness, lethargy, hypotension and slow heart rate. The interaction of Valerian with other drugs is not known and long term use of Valerian during pregnancy is discouraged. (10)

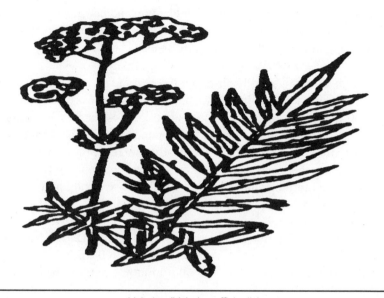

Valerian (Valerian officinalis)

HORMONES

Melatonin is a naturally occuring hormone produced in the pineal gland of human brains. Melatonin is structurally similar to serotonin. It is important in regulating sleep and our circadian rhythm; the normal 24 hour biological clock in the human body. Melatonin secretion decreases with age and is believed to responsible for chronic insomnia common in many elderly patients. (11)

One study in elderly insomniacs with significantly lower blood levels of melatonin than elderly patients with normal sleep patterns, showed that melatonin supplementation decreased the time required to fall asleep and sustained sleep maintenance. (12) In another double blind controlled study of 12 patients who complained of chronic insomnia, the melatonin treated group showed improved sleep onset, sleep quality and duration. (13) In another study, melatonin was compared to a benzodiazepine drug halcion. Unlike halcion, melatonin did not affect the autonomic nervous system and did not suppress REM (rapid eye movement) sleep. Melatonin appears to be safe and effective for the treatment of insomnia for many individuals. (14,15)

Other beneficial effects of melatonin include jet lag, delayed sleep phase syndrome, use in shift workers, immunostimulant properties, anti-aging and anti-cancer effects. (116, 17)

Melatonin is readily absorbed through the digestive system and has a relatively short half-life. Peak blood melatonin levels occur within 30 to 60 minutes following oral consumption. Melatonin is virtually non-toxic and oral doses of up to several hundred milligrams have been given to laboratory animals without adverse reactions. Some side effects include headache, stomach upset, nausea, depression, feeling drowsy in the morning and a "heavy head." It's use during pregnancy is strongly discouraged. (11)

Oral consumption of melatonin should mimic the body's natural production of this hormone. A dose of 0.5 to 6.0 milligrams in the evening approximately 30 to 60 minutes before bedtime is recommended.

RECOMMENDATIONS: Daily unless otherwise stated

Myo-inositol..500 mg
Niacinamide...1 gram
Humulus lupulus (4:1)...300 mg
Passiflora incarnata (5:1)..150 mg
Valerian officinalis (4:1)..400 mg

REFERENCES

(1) Shirlow MJ et al: A study of caffeine consumption and symptoms. Int. J. Epidemiol. 14(2):239-48, 1985
(2) Stone BM: Sleep and low doses of alcohol. Electroencephalogr. Clin. Neurophysiol. 48(6):706-9, 1980
(3) Pfeiffer C: Mental and Elemental Nutrients. New Canaan, Conn., Keats Publishing Company, 1975
(4) Mohler H et al: Nicotinamide is a brain constituent with benzodiazepine-like actions. Nature 278:563-65, 1979

(5)   Hartmann EL speaking at a symposium sponsored by the AMA - quoted in Clin. Psychiat. News, March 1985

(6)   Leung AY: Encyclopedia of Common Natural Ingredients Used in Food, Drugs, and Cosmetics. John Wiley & Sons, New York, NY, 1980

(7)   Wohlfart R et al: Planta Medica 48:120, 1983

(8)   Lawrence Review of Natural Products. JB Lippincott Company, St. Louis, Missouri, May 1989

(9)   Lawrence Review of Natural Products. JB Lippincott Company, St Louis, Missouri, Feb. 1986

(10) Hobbs C: Valerian. Herbal/Gram 21: 19-34, Fall 1989

(11) Cupp MJ: Melatonin. American Family Physician, 1421-25, October, 1997

(12) Haimov I et al: Melatonin replacement therapy of elderly insomniacs. Sleep. 18:598-603, 1995

(13) Garfinkel D et al: Improvement of sleep quality in elderly people by controlled-release melatonin. Lancet. 346:541-4, 1995

(14) Zhdanova IV et al: Sleep-inducing effects of low doses of melatonin ingested in the evening. Clin. Pharmacol. Ther. 57:552-8, 1995

(15) Ferini-Strambi L et al: Triazolam and melatonin effects on cardiac autonomic function during sleep. Clin. Neuropharmacol. 18:405-9, 1995

(16) Melatonin: The Lawrence Review of Natural Products. St. Louis: Facts and Comparisons, January, 1996

(17) Petrie K et al: Effect of melatonin on jet lag after long haul flights. BMJ. 298:705-7, 1989

(18) Hofbrauer LC and Heufelder AE: Endocrinology meets immunology: T-lymphocytes as novel targets for melatonin. Eur. J. Endocrinol. 134:424-25, 1996

INDEX